Why  ...ling?

A compariso... ...e science and efficacy of natural healing with that of pharmaceuticals

Fletcher Kovich, Lic.Ac.

CuriousPages Publishing
Bristol, United Kingdom

Published 2021 by CuriousPages Publishing, Bristol, UK

Copyright © 2021 Fletcher Kovich

The author asserts his moral right under the Copyright, Designs and Patents Act, 1988, to be identified as the author of this work.
All Rights reserved. No part of this publication may be reproduced, copied, stored in a retrieval system, or transmitted, in any form or by any means, without the prior written consent of the copyright holder, nor be otherwise circulated in any form of binding or cover other than that in which it is published and without a similar condition being imposed on the subsequent purchaser.

ISBN 978-1-3999-0182-6 (paperback)

This book does not serve as a manual on how to do acupuncture or acupressure. Such treatments, whether by needling, moxibustion, cupping or pressure, should always be performed by a qualified Chinese Medicine acupuncturist.

Preface

This book is aimed at the general reader. The book relies on sound, scientific research, and on a detailed analytical study of the ancient Chinese medicine classics, by a practitioner (myself) with many years of clinical experience of traditional Chinese acupuncture, and also a background in the sciences.

All controversial content related to mainstream healthcare includes references to the source material. However, the main material relating to Chinese medicine is not usually referenced, since the book does not intend to prove this material, but merely to report it. If you would like to know more about the evidence that this aspect of the book is based on, the full detail is provided in the textbook: *Acupuncture Today and in Ancient China*, by Fletcher Kovich. This book describes all the evidence in detail, and provides references to all the source material.

Contents

Preface 3
1. Introduction 7
2. What is Chinese Medicine? 9
    How an accurate diagnosis is made 14
    How our thoughts and emotions are produced by our organs 16
    How people become ill 25
3. The pharmaceutical approach to healthcare 31
    How drugs are designed 33
    What is the whole "blood pressure" issue about? 33
    What are the common types of drugs used? 37
4. How does natural healing treat "blood pressure" issues? .. 49
    The approach of mainstream healthcare 53
5. The conduct of drug companies 61
    Serious harms concealed, purely for profit 62
    Pushing drugs for non-approved uses 72
    Defrauding taxpayers and bribing doctors 75
    To sell their products, drug companies routinely use bribery and covering up of serious adverse effects 76
6. Can the reported outcome of a drug trial be taken at face value? 79
    Why are drugs designed for one purpose but often marketed for many other purposes? 84
    Other dishonest methods used to manipulate drug trials to produce misleading results 84
7. How are useless and harmful drugs pushed? 89
    First, produce a fraudulent trial 89
    Then, bribe the doctors 89
    Negative data about drugs is concealed to make the drugs seem effective 92
8. Drug companies create fictitious illnesses to boost profits 101
    The madness of psychiatry 104
9. An outsider's assessment of mainstream healthcare 111

10. Do vaccines work? 123
    The theory of vaccination 129
    How might vaccines cause autoimmune conditions? 131
    The other toxic aspect of vaccines 136
    The war on "germs", an alternative view 140

11. How do we become ill? 145

12. Why has an inept, misguided system been adopted by mainstream healthcare? 157

13. What is the value of a diagnosis from mainstream healthcare? 175

    References and endnotes 191
    Index 209
    Further reading 215

1. Introduction

Because of the way the drug industry has developed, the pharmaceutical approach to healthcare is not now capable of healing. But rather it prevents healing from happening, and only harms the patient's long-term health.

To devotees of mainstream healthcare, this might seem a puzzling statement. But this book clearly explains why this is the case. It describes the ideas behind drug design; the flaws in these ideas; it explains why this approach is not capable of healing; and it provides the unvarnished facts about the fraudulent techniques used by drug companies to conceal the harms in their drugs and falsely claim they are effective—all in the pursuit of profit and to the detriment of healthcare. Such a fraudulent system has now become state sponsored, worldwide—due mainly to commercial concerns.

Today's mainstream healthcare can best be regarded as a medical religion. All its ideas are believed by the majority of people and repeated as though factual and unquestionable. But many of these ideas are misguided, unscientific, and certainly do not produce effective treatments but rather "treatments" that only impede a patient's health.

This is because most of the commonly used drugs are designed to chemically block the normal function of healthy aspects of the body, in an attempt to conceal symptoms, simply because this is an easy thing for the pharmaceutical industry to do, and many billions can be made from doing this. But because this approach is so detrimental to healthcare, many arguments have been developed by the drug industry to conceal the facts and mislead doctors, the media and public. These arguments are now taught to doctors in medical schools, and accepted by them. Hence the media, politicians and the public (whose information comes from doctors) are all equally mislead.

Because this misinformation is so all pervasive in society today, to be able to properly understand the true nature of the drug-based approach to healthcare, it is necessary to first understand how natural

Why Use Natural Healing?

healing works. This then puts the drug-based approach in context and enables it to be seen objectively, when all its obvious flaws then become apparent.

This book therefore begins with a clear description of how Chinese medicine (with over 2,000 years of consistent clinical results) uses a natural communication system in our body to return our main organs to normal function, which then clears the symptoms of our illness. With each main organ, the book describes all the possible symptoms that result when the organ malfunctions, and how acupuncture is used to correct these subtle organ malfunctions and hence clear the related symptoms. It also describes how our thoughts are able to disrupt our organ functions, which is the most common cause of illness today.

The pharmaceutical approach is then described. This includes how drugs are designed, their intended purpose, and the actual effect they have (the treatment of blood-pressure related issues is taken as an example). The flaws in this approach are clearly described, and many examples are given of the fraud that drug companies now routinely use to cover up the harms in their drugs, and to make untrue claims for the effectiveness of them, by rigging drug trials and fraudulently massaging data.

Being able to view all this from the perspective of natural healing, makes it possible to clearly see how today's drug approach is misguided from its conception, and how it can only block the normal function of a patient's main organs, preventing them from ever enjoying good health.

Once these facts are realized, and you can see beyond the propaganda, the sad reality becomes evident. The world is now trapped into not having a real healthcare system, and using one that is only detrimental to world health. But facing these sad facts is a precursor to achieving real healthcare for all.

2. What is Chinese Medicine?

Chinese medicine and acupuncture was fully documented in a series of scrolls by separate authors, called the *Nei Jing*, dating back to around the 2nd century BC.

In general, it was not felt necessary to give names to the conditions that people suffered. Instead, it was recognised that when one of the main organs was stressed in any way, this produced a range of possible symptoms in the patient. For example, when the pancreas function was poor, it was found that this could produce any combination of the following symptoms:

- a poor appetite (prefer to only eat small amounts);
- general weakness (and hence the tendency to avoid speaking), and feeling tired after eating;
- abdominal bloating and discomfort (particularly after eating), excess gas, frequent loose stools; intolerances for certain foods, such as dairy or wheat;
- poor sense of taste; cravings for sweet food;
- muscles of the limbs are weak and soft (emaciated);
- tendency to bruise easily or have mild haemorrhages or purple spots or patches on the skin, blood in the stools, excessive menstrual flow or bleeding of the uterus;
- feeling a bearing-down sensation in the abdomen, possibly with prolapse of the anus or of internal organs such as the stomach, kidneys, uterus or bladder;
- pain or discomfort anywhere along the pancreas or stomach meridian; and
- the tendency to be always thinking.

Why Use Natural Healing?

To alleviate these symptoms, the pancreas was treated, so that it returned to normal function, which then caused all the related symptoms to clear.

One way of treating a particular organ was by using combinations of herbs that had been found to affect that organ. But another, novel way was as follows.

It was discovered that each of our organs resonated with a particular path around the surface of our body. These paths are known today as meridians. When a particular organ was stressed, this caused locations on that organ's meridian to also be similarly stressed, which caused the location to feel tender when pressed, or for the skin to be reddened, or to feel warm, or for anomalies, such as boils to appear there. In some cases, aching or even shooting pains could occur along a particular organ's meridian for the same reason (that is, to reflect a particular type of malfunction in that organ).

When any of these affected locations on an organ's meridian were stimulated, this caused the local stress to clear from that tissue, and because of the resonance between this location and the related organ, this also caused that organ to release its stress. The organ function returned to normal (often within a few seconds), and this caused the related symptoms to clear.

The stimulation was achieved either by massage, by applying heat, or by using fine needles. This latter option is known today as acupuncture.

The symptoms related to the other main organs

When the liver function is stagnated, this could produce any of the following symptoms:

- discomfort at the front or back of the torso at the level of the liver (the hypochondrium), frequent sighing or hiccupping;
- feeling of irritability, with outbursts of angry shouting;
- muscular spasms, cramps, twitching, stiff neck;
- a feeling as though something were stuck in your throat;

- fluctuations of mood, melancholy or depression, paranoia;
- migraines or headaches with pain on the top or sides of the head or associated with the eyes, visual disturbances;
- dizziness, vertigo, hearing high pitch ringing sounds (tinnitus), insomnia;
- strong pain, stiffness or discomfort anywhere along the liver or gallbladder meridian, particularly on the head, neck, hips, and outside of the legs;
- effects on other organs, producing constipation, or the alternation of constipation with loose stools and other digestive signs;
- (in women) irregular periods with cramps, tender breasts, either scanty or absent menses or, alternatively, heavy flow with clots, and emotional fluctuations and irritability in the pre-menstrual phase (PMS); and (in all patients)
- the tendency to be controlling.

When the kidney function is poor, this could produce any of the following symptoms (note that when the "kidneys" are mentioned in Chinese Medicine, this also includes the adrenal glands and the sex organs, all considered as a single organ):

- soreness and weakness of the lower back (lumbar region), and weak knees or stiff joints;
- frequent and urgent urination (it cannot be put off), and dribbling of urine after urination, or incontinence (enuresis);
- premature ejaculation in men;
- hay fever and other allergies, frequent colds and flu;
- dizziness or lightheaded feeling (particularly after sex in men);
- oedema, particularly in the lower half of the body;
- low-pitch tinnitus (or rumbling or swishing sounds);
- deafness or being hard of hearing;
- loss of balance;
- tendency to feel fearful;
- craving salty food;

Why Use Natural Healing?

- shortness of breath, asthma (where it is difficult to breathe in);
- insomnia;
- poor short term memory;
- thirst, afternoon fever (hot flushes) and night sweating, dry mouth, hot hands and feet;
- cold limbs, aversion to cold;
- low energy and apathy;
- slow physical development, poor skeletal development, brittle bones, poorly formed or loose teeth;
- slow mental development;
- mental dullness, premature senility, dementia;
- premature greying and hair loss; and
- impotence, or infertility.

When the lung function is poor, this could produce any of the following symptoms:

- shortness of breath which is worse on exertion;
- weak cough with clear, thin sputum;
- poor energy and pale complexion, with an even greater energy lag between three and five p.m.;
- lack of desire to talk, having a quiet voice, and tiring quickly when having to talk a lot;
- spontaneous daytime sweating;
- frequently suffering colds and flu, and generally being easily affected by external pathogens;
- tendency to feel the cold and having a dislike of being in the wind or cold;
- a poor sense of smell, blocked nose, and sinuses; and
- pain or discomfort anywhere along the lung or large intestine meridian.

And when the heart function is poor, this could produce any of the following symptoms. Note that some of these symptoms are similar to those produced by the lungs; only when the lungs are affected, a cough is present; whereas when the heart is affected, palpitations are present:

- palpitations (awareness of heartbeat);
- shortness of breath on exertion;
- spontaneous sweating;
- lethargy;
- a weak pulse;
- anxiety, panic attacks, restlessness, unease;
- being easily startled by noises or anything unexpected in the immediate environment;
- speech defects such as stammering or stuttering; dyslexia;
- poor long-term memory;
- dream-disturbed sleep;
- insomnia (hard to fall asleep);
- stuffiness or stabbing pains in the chest, which may radiate to the left shoulder and arm;
- possibly also a blue-purple tinge to the face, lips and nails;
- muttering to oneself;
- depression or mental dullness;
- introverted manner, unable to make eye contact;
- incessant or incoherent talking;
- violent behaviour (hitting or scolding people);
- laughing and crying without reason;
- paranoia, hysteria, mental confusion;
- aphasia (partial loss of the ability to communicate with words);
- loss of consciousness (sudden collapse or coma);
- chills, cold limbs; a blue tinge to the lips;
- profuse sweating;
- feeble breathing;
- feeble and fading pulse; and
- mental "cloudiness" or even coma.

Why Use Natural Healing?

As can be seen from the above lists, the range of symptoms associated with some of the organs can be extensive, and covers symptoms in many areas, including our thoughts and emotions as well as the physical symptoms. In the accompanying book, *Acupuncture Today and in Ancient China*, it is clearly explained why and how these symptoms are produced by the related organ. Once this is understood, it can be appreciated how treating the five main organs with traditional acupuncture can have a wide-ranging and deep effect on a person's health, including the mental and emotional aspects of their personality.

How an accurate diagnosis is made

The process of making a diagnosis often begins by asking the patient questions about the symptoms they have. The intention is to identify any of the symptoms from the above lists. Some of the symptoms could be produced by more than one organ, and in this case, further questions are asked to identify the organ concerned. When about three symptoms, or more, have been identified that could be produced by a single organ, then that organ is considered to be stressed. This diagnosis would then be confirmed by examining the patient's tongue, and taking their pulses.

Tongue examination

Many patterns can be seen on the tongue that can accurately indicate which organ or organs are stressed. Particular areas of the tongue relate to certain organs, and when that organ is stressed, this produces redness in that area; or the area may be more or less swollen than the surrounding area; or the tongue coating may be affected, in either its colour or thickness. As well as the area of these anomalies indicating which organ is involved, the type of the anomaly also indicates the type of malfunction in the organ.

A common example is a tongue that is generally swollen, usually accompanied by teeth marks on the side. This indicates that the person's pancreas function is weak. In my clinical experience, a person with such a tongue would also be a heavy thinker or worrier. There is a clear link between over thinking and poor pancreas function.

Interestingly, babies are usually born with a weak digestion (perhaps because these organs were not used prior to birth). And this explains why a baby's tongue is usually swollen, indicating that their pancreas function is weak (the pancreas being the main digestive organ).

Another common condition in developed countries is stress. The symptoms of stress are usually produced by a person's liver and gallbladder; and the function of these organs is usually impeded when certain thought patterns are blocked (such as when we become aware of rules being broken, or things being unjust, unfair, or wrong for some other reason). The left and right sides of the tongue relate to the liver and gallbladder. When someone's liver is heavily affected by this type of stress, the sides of their tongue would appear reddened.

The organ "pulses"

When the "pulses" are taken in Chinese Medicine, this is entirely different to the process of taking a person's pulse in mainstream healthcare.

In Chinese Medicine, the practitioner takes the pulses in three different locations on each wrist; and due to the relationships between the practitioners fingers (which each have different meridians terminating on them) and the left or right side of the patient, this causes the shape of the pulses under each of the practitioner's fingers to adopt a pattern that pertains to a particular organ. The pulse felt in each position can indicate the strength of that organ's function, and also the type of any malfunction.

There is usually an extremely reliable correlation between these patterns, the tongue diagnosis, and also the symptoms that the patient experiences. These methods in combination usually produce an accurate diagnosis. But there are still other ways that the practitioner can confirm the diagnosis.

Meridian locations

Another method commonly used is to examine the meridians at key locations. When each of the main organs is stressed, it is usual for key locations along the organ's related meridian to also have anomalies. The location (a key acupuncture point for that organ) would usually feel tender when pressed. This is an extremely reliable diagnostic indicator. But there may also be other signs, such as the skin being reddened, or feeling warmer or cooler than the surrounding skin, or for anomalies such as boils or eruptions to appear.

All these different methods provide a whole range of diagnostic techniques that can reliably confirm that the problem lies with a particular organ. And all these methods rely only on the skill of the practitioner; there are no machines or devices needed to make an accurate, reliable diagnosis.

Other signs that assist a diagnosis

The knowledge and experience of the practitioner can also provide other techniques to confirm the diagnosis. When a person's health is dominated by the malfunction of a particular organ, this causes the patient to adopt certain mental and emotional patterns, and also other reliable indicators, such as their tone of voice, complexion, and the way they move.

For example, when a person's health is dominated by their liver function being stagnated, the person would tend to be over controlling. They would be forever straightening objects or tidying up; and they would insist that things were done in a certain way, and if any of these "rules" of theirs were broken, they would find this extremely irritating, to the point where they could frequently erupt in angry outbursts (or if they suppressed their anger, this could lead to migraines or crippling pains along the gallbladder meridian). Their voice would also be notably loud. When they were simply conversing routinely, it would sound as though they were shouting. These signs are a reliable indicator of stagnated liver function.

Similar patterns exist with the pancreas, kidneys, lungs and heart.

How our thoughts and emotions are produced by our organs

In ancient China it was recognized that certain thought patterns resembled the physical function of certain organs, and that when those thought patterns became unhealthy, this affected the physical function of the related organ.

From this, and much other related evidence, it seems probable that as we evolved, and our thoughts gradually became more complex, the physical functions of our organs were utilized to process our thoughts. Because the "brain matter" related to our organ functions had already existed for perhaps millions of years before we started having more complex thoughts, it would clearly have been easier and quicker for our conscious mind to utilize this existing brain matter, rather than creating new "logic circuits" to do this new job. This pattern exists not only in humans, but also in all other creatures.

The effects on our liver function

For example, the physical function of our liver is to organize the flow of physical substances around our body; the production and supply of energy in our body; and to creatively draw on different resources to best meet the current needs of our body. And in our thoughts, our mind utilizes these same liver functions to organize the world around us, to work out how to best do each task, and to produce creative solutions to problems. The behaviour this produces in us is to be constantly organizing ourselves and the people around us. In some people, their personality has become dominated by their liver function, and this would cause other people to view their behaviour as being over controlling.

This connection between our organ functions and thoughts always works in both directions. And when our liver-related thoughts are blocked (by something being out of place, or a person not behaving as they should; that is, the way we would like them to), this causes our liver function to become blocked, or stagnated. Our liver feels that the substances in our body have been blocked from flowing normally. This is a serious situation for our body, and this causes our liver to produce that feeling of anger or rage that we immediately feel. Our "blood starts to boil." This is the feeling of our physical liver trying to move the blocked substances.

Due to social constraints, we would usually suppress our anger or irritation, to some degree. Some people are better than others at concealing their irritation. But the people whose personality is heavily influenced by their liver would soon find it impossible to contain their building rage and may start shouting to attempt to get their will obeyed. They may even resort to physical violence to remedy this "wrong" behaviour in other people, or in inanimate objects. Things such as computer software or gadgets may often not perform as we would like, and there are less social constraints governing how we treat such devices, therefore we might frequently find ourselves indulging in outbursts of rage when software or gadgets do not behave in the way we expect.

If we are more "self controlled," and suppress most of these instances, the resulted suppression of the physical function of our liver can lead to serious and painful conditions, such as migraines, depression, and many other conditions due to the blocked flow of the substances in our body, or the production of our energy.

All the above effects are related to stress, which is basically the improper behaviour of other people and institutions, particularly in a work environment. And the fact that we are compelled to continue suffering a stressful job, is in itself yet one more injustice (in other words, the breaking of a "rule", as far as our liver function is concerned; "it's not fair that I have to endure this; this is part of my work, so I must endure being treated this way, otherwise I may lose my job and starve").

When a person behaves in any of these ways, this is a reliable indicator that their liver function is stagnated, and the existence of these patterns can also help to confirm the diagnosis.

The effects on our pancreas function

Another common cause of disease in developed societies is over thinking. This affects our pancreas function, and produces the symptoms of "IBS".

The pancreas is our body's main digestive organ, and our mind uses this function to digest our thoughts. The functions of all the organs vary throughout the day, in a 24 hour cycle. With the pancreas, its function peaks at eleven a.m. And people with poor pancreas function find that they can only think clearly before about midday, which reinforces the connection between the pancreas function and thinking. But in a developed society, we are usually required to be thinking all day long. If our work does not involve thinking, people whose personality is dominated by their pancreas would be thinking all day long anyway, worrying about life, or just simply making up things to think about.

Because of the two-way link between an organ's physical functions and the mental application of those functions, when we think all day, it is as though our pancreas were having to digest a banquet of food all day long; and our pancreas becomes tired. It can then no longer properly digest *any* physical food, and this produces the symptoms of "IBS", including loose stools, abdominal bloating and discomfort, and any of the other symptoms listed on page 9.

What makes this situation worse, is that the problems we mull over, either related to our work or social life, are usually hard to solve (hard to digest). Again, due to this two-way link between our processing of such thoughts and our physical pancreas function, the effect of this is to transform all our physical food into food that is hard to digest. Therefore, not only is our lifestyle constantly weakening our pancreas function, but it is also tricking our pancreas into regarding all the *physical* food we eat as being hard to digest, making the situation worse.

Diagnostically, there is a reliable link between over thinking and poor pancreas function. In my clinical experience, a patient with poor pancreas function always has a swollen tongue and is constantly thinking or worrying. These three things always go hand in hand.

The effect on our heart function

In our body, our heart's function is to "reach out" to the other organs and bodily tissue and spread nourishment to them, via the network of arteries and veins. When this function is used by our mind, this produces our desire to reach out to the people around us. This is most commonly achieved through speech, but we also use touch and eye contact. And our heart's function also produces in us the desire to help others and the ability to be able to empathise with them.

Our sense of speech is heavily influenced by our heart. When our heart function is poor, this often produces speech defects, such as stammering or stuttering. This effect can be seen instantly in many people whose heart function may otherwise be normal. When they momentarily adopt a position that they know is immoral, such as when lying or treating a person unfairly (which only applies to people who have an awareness of morality) this will momentarily weaken their heart function, which in turn affects their speech and produces a momentary stammer or stutter.

When we do reach out and help someone, because we are acting on this desire that our heart function has produced, this enhances that function, and the "warm glow" that we feel in our heart is a reflection of this. Our heart feels energized, feels momentarily stronger.

Conversely, most societies usually encourage men to "not complain", to not share their emotional concerns, to "take it like a man" and just keep quiet and suffer in silence. In effect, society encourages men to live a lonely existence. When men do this, they are undermining their heart's desire to reach out to others. And due to the two-way link between an organ's physical and mental functions, this weakens their physical heart. They are undermining their own heart, and in time this could result in diseased arteries or even a heart attack. Their social connections are diseased, therefore their physical arteries become diseased (which are the heart's "social" connections with the other organs around it).

This conditioning starts in early childhood. And another social situation in our early life that can result in poor heart function is when a child has poor social connections with their family. In other words, when there are poor family relationships. Since our speech is heavily associated with our heart function, this situation would tend to produce speech defects, such as stammering or stuttering. And while a person's heart retains this poor function into their later life, this would also tend to produce "faulty social connections" in them. They would tend to behave and talk in ways that seem strange, would often make inappropriate comments, and may be constantly smiling inappropriately and talking with an amused tone of voice.

As a practitioner of Chinese Medicine, these signs provide another reliable diagnostic device. In some cases, it is often possible for a practitioner to make an accurate diagnosis merely from the sound of a person's voice. Of course, the diagnosis would then be confirmed by using all the other methods.

The effect on our kidney function

When we refer to the "kidneys" in Chinese Medicine, this means three organs in combination: the kidneys, the adrenal glands, and the sex organs. All the other organs have their own dedicated meridian, but with these three organs, they share a single meridian, which is known as the kidney meridian. And when stimulating this one meridian, this treats all these three organs at once. Therefore, from the physiological point of view, it is likely that these three separate structures should be more correctly considered to be separate parts of the same organ.

In our body, the functions of these organs (in combination) are mainly concerned with our self-preservation, both in the present and the future. Amongst other functions, the "kidneys" coordinate our growth and development, from conception through to adulthood; are the key reproductive organ, being responsible for fertility and our sexual behaviour, which thus provides us with our engagement in life and the desire to go on. They regulate the body's energy usage, so as to ensure the proper function of all the organs, thus enabling us to function at our best in the present and also enabling us to deal with stressful situations; and they manage and support the immunity.

Hence, when the kidney function is poor, a person may have low libido, a lack of drive or enthusiasm for life, and may seem to be living in slow motion. Our kidney function tends to weaken in old age, which would produce all these symptoms which are familiar in most old people. But these same symptoms can occur in us if our kidney function becomes poor in earlier life.

When any of our kidney-related concerns are undermined, the kidneys produce the emotion of fear, usually accompanied by an adrenaline surge, to prompt us to remedy the threat to our survival. The threat might be simply the undermining of our status or position;

it does not have to be a threat of physical violence. Insecurity is another common threat. From our kidneys' point of view, this threatens the survival of our body, which is one of its main concerns. Therefore, when we feel constant insecurity, or fear, this undermines our kidney's concerns, which in turn undermines our kidney function, and this may produce any of the symptoms listed on page 11.

In our modern world, such insecurities are common. People may fear losing their job, or constantly worry about being able to pay bills. Or they may fear losing a relationship if they do not work hard in ways that they cannot really understand. Any of these concerns may then cause them to be constantly running on adrenaline, to try to perform better; and this state itself also weakens the kidneys. The adrenaline surge is meant as an emergency measure, to enable us to cope with a short term threat. But when we live almost constantly in that state, the overuse of this emergency measure also weakens our kidney function, which again may produce any of the symptoms listed on page 11.

Another common health problem related to the mental aspect of the kidneys is when our spirit is defeated. The kidney "logic" identifies our goals in life, our ambitions, and fosters our ideas about our worth, status, or position in life; and the kidneys then drive us to achieve these ambitions. But when any of our ambitions are defeated, or our status or position in life is taken away, this undermines these kidney functions in our thoughts, which then also undermines and hence impedes the kidneys' physical function.

In this situation, the person's "spark" would be clearly diminished; they would become gloomy, dispirited. The kidney function of regulating the production of energy would become poor and consequently the other main organs would function poorly. The person would become sluggish, would certainly be melancholic or in a depressive state (as though their body had been shut down) and they may feel like giving up on life, having no drive or spirit.

Because acupuncture directly prompts the organs to return to normal function, this can also immediately correct the mental aspect of an organ; and there are some key kidney acupoints that can produce impressive, instant results in people whose "spirit" has taken a hard knock. At the end of the treatment, the person can seem to have suddenly come to life, with the spark having returned to their eyes, and they can suddenly look years younger.

The effect on our Lung function

The physical function of the lungs could be summarized as: to take in something intangible (air) from outside, sort the good from the bad, incorporate the precious (the oxygen) and let go of the waste (the carbon dioxide). And when our mind uses this function to process our thoughts, this enables us to discern quality in the intangible things around us.

People who tend to overuse the mental aspect of their lung function become perfectionists. But the more we look for perfection, the less we are able to find it, which creates a constant feeling of disappointment. And when this lung function is frustrated in our thoughts, this failure is duplicated in the *physical* lung function, which weakens it. Therefore, this group of people would usually appear sad and have a weak lung function.

The lungs are also weakened due to grief. Grief is not only felt due to the loss of a loved one, but can also be felt due to the loss of anything the person cherishes, such as their job, career, social status, material possessions or wealth, and so on. This may be because the lung function of "letting go of the waste" is now challenged and resisted by our conscious mind, which in turn weakens the lungs.

Another factor that can lead to poor lung function is overuse of your voice. In Chinese medicine, it is recognised that one function of the lungs is to support the voice. When the lung function is weakened by illness, this can often result in the voice failing. Conversely, overuse of the voice tends to weaken the lung function.

In my practice I have treated many teachers and almost all of them had health issues related to poor lung function. Teachers not only must use their voice excessively, and often project it over a resistant and vocal class of children; but also the defensive aspect of their lungs is continuously taxed due to the prevalence of colds amongst children, and also the fact that teachers can sometimes feel "under attack" by their students—which has the same effect on us that physical pathogens do and would certainly also tax the immunity. Their lungs would also be taxed due to them having to constantly assess the quality of their students' work (teachers, by definition, are perfectionists), which also tends to weaken the lungs.

Another symptom that reflects the prevalence of lung issues amongst teachers is the fact that many teachers tend to suffer an energy lag around three p.m. This is the time of day when the lung function is at its weakest, hence the energy lag felt by people with poor lung function. This energy lag, along with any other signs and symptoms related to poor lung function (as listed on page 12), tends to clear after a few treatments (which I mention to demonstrate that this energy lag is not merely due to the fact that three p.m. is near the end of most teachers' working day).

Treating the mental factors

The lungs also actively expel the waste product of respiration (carbon dioxide), and when the lung function is used to process our thoughts, this ability enables us to let go of "waste". That is, anything in our life that may have become harmful to us. This is often something we once cherished but has now become harmful, such as relationships that have gone bad, projects we started that are not now working. But when a person's lung function is poor, this also weakens their ability to let go of this "waste" in their life. Another facet of this function is that they may bear grudges long after other people would have forgotten about the issue and moved on.

When a person is trapped in such a pattern of mental activity, it can be extremely difficult to break the pattern. But one of the strengths of acupuncture is that it prompts the physical organs to return to normal function and does this without involving our conscious mind. In effect, acupuncture seems to "get under the radar" of our conscious mind. And once the organ functions are normalized, this tends to also normalize each organ's mental functions; and after a few treatments patients often describe the changes they have spontaneously adopted in their mental behaviour.

For a fuller discussion of the mental aspects of our organ functions, see the textbook: *Acupuncture Today and in Ancient China*, by Fletcher Kovich.

How people become ill

Because the functions of our main organs are utilized by our mind to process our thoughts and produce our emotions, when a particular thought pattern or emotion becomes inappropriate, this disrupts the physical function of the related organ, which can then produce serious physical symptoms.

Liver-related symptoms are often the most powerful, such as migraines, period cramps, muscular pains, sciatica or neuralgia (see page 10); and the mental/emotional symptoms related to the liver function can be just as powerful, such as constant rage, paranoia, or depression. But the other main organs can also produce overpowering symptoms, such as the kidney-related low back ache, feelings of fear and insecurity, impotence, lack of motivation or engagement in life (page 11); and the pancreas-related IBS and constant over thinking and worrying, often without being able to arrive at satisfactory conclusions (circular thought patterns).

The above process gives our mind (and the society we live in) the ability to disrupt the physical function of our organs, which then produces our illness. Hence, most of the physical symptoms we suffer have usually been created by our own thought patterns (which includes the way our mind reacts to the society we live in). In my clinical experience, most long term, serious conditions that people suffer have such an underlying cause.

This detailed knowledge of the interaction between our thoughts, emotions, and our physical organ functions, is beyond the understanding so far reached by today's mainstream medics. To them, this is counter intuitive. They imagine the brain is a separate, all powerful computer; whereas the ancient Chinese realized that our organs play the dominant role in determining our personality and health. Why does this ancient knowledge seem so much more advanced than today's mainstream medical thinking?

The ancient approach to healthcare

The knowledge of the ancient Chinese physicians was built up over centuries using a simple approach. The "meridian system" consists of specific tracts of tissue on the body that are affected when the related organs are stressed. When a person was ill, they had a range of symptoms, and also a particular meridian would be affected (having tender locations, or other anomalies along that particular tract of tissue). Knowledge of this system enabled the physicians to build up detailed knowledge about the symptoms that result when each organ is stressed in some way (as listed on pages 9 to 13).

It was only necessary to know what symptoms are produced when a particular organ was stressed; they did not need to know the microscopic detail of *how* these symptoms resulted or were produced in the body (and those symptoms could be physical, mental or emotional). Knowledge of this whole range of symptoms was gained, covering just about every common state that people could suffer. And because they knew which organ was malfunctioning to produce the particular symptoms, they could use this same "meridian system" to correct the organ's function and return the patient to good health.

When an organ is malfunctioning, this causes anomalies to occur at particular locations on that organ's related meridian, and stimulating those same locations, encourages the organ to return to normal function. This happens within a few seconds, and the patient returns to good health, until the factors in society that made them ill in the first place, are re-established, and the same organ malfunctions recur.

The great power of this healing system lies in its simplicity, and also in the fact that the physician does not *need* to know how the body works at the microscopic level, and does not even *want* to know. The chemical communication between the organs and the body is corrected by the organs themselves, which is as it should be; after all, the *organs* are the experts on their own chemistry.

This approach not only produced a powerful healing system, but it also enabled the ancient Chinese to understand common and important mechanisms in the body that are not yet understood by today's mainstream healthcare. This includes the cause of IBS; the underlying cause of most cases of asthma and allergies such as hay fever; and also the mechanism that produces all the symptoms of stress, and the details of the mental cause and how this affects the liver function, which is the organ that produces all the symptoms. Also a wide range of common mental issues are also clearly understood.

However, apart from conditions with powerful symptoms, other conditions that can sometimes seem intangible are also routinely treated with acupuncture.

Patient Example

Female, aged 45. I initially treated this patient for migraines, and she also wished to stop using various pharmaceuticals. She responded well to treatment and her health was transformed. But because she was under a lot of stress in her life, she then continued attending clinic for a monthly maintenance treatment, to retain the good health she had regained. In this one treatment, a lot of emotional stress had built up over the past month. This affected her periods, producing a few days of PMS (which was now unusual for her), notably tender breasts, some muscular cramps, and in the session she was uncharacteristically emotional. Yet, the other diagnostic signs were subtle. Her organ "pulses" were affected (particularly kidney, lungs, heart and liver), and key acupoints were notably tender (lung-1, kidney-1; and liver-3 was very tender).

Ordinarily none of these states would have been seen as unusual by mainstream medics, and would certainly not have shown up in any of their usual diagnostic tests. But in the acupuncture treatment, she responded quickly; her organ pulses returned to normal, the tender meridian locations diminished greatly, and at the end of the session she felt much calmer and relaxed. She had been treated on a deep level, simply by returning her main organs to normal function. After this, and her other routine acupuncture sessions, she usually felt emotionally and physically much improved, almost like a new person.

There is no doubt that this type of treatment makes a real difference to the functions of a patient's main organs, and this is a good example of what Chinese acupuncture does.

Yet these kinds of organ "malfunctions" build up gradually, over weeks, months or even years, so the patient does not usually notice how ill they are. If they are experiencing strong symptoms, then of course they notice those, but they usually remain unaware of their general state of stress, until, that is, their organ functions are returned to normal with acupuncture. At this instant, patients often describe the feeling as euphoric. But this euphoric state is simply normality; and it only feels this good to them because they were used to feeling constantly stressed. Yet today's mainstream healthcare is much less sensitive, and in these types of situation it would usually not even be able to detect a problem with the patient's organ functions.

Today's approach to healthcare

In contrast, today's approach is to study the body at the microscopic level and attempt to work out how it works. When a person is ill, and symptoms appear, the physicians then attempt to directly intervene themselves (usually focussed only on the symptom). This might be by attempting to block an aspect of the body's chemistry, or repair or replace "broken" or "worn out" parts, or even replacing a whole "irrevocably diseased" organ.

Due to the limitations of drug design, and of physiology knowledge, today's healthcare is not able to treat an organ directly to return it to normal function, as in the above Chinese acupuncture examples. And anyway, mainstream healthcare is not even able to detect these "routine" organ malfunctions—to the sensitive degree that Chinese medicine can; it can only detect an organ malfunction when it has become so extreme that the organ has almost ceased to function. Instead, mainstream healthcare has focussed on chemically blocking the normal, healthy function of some aspect of the body, in an attempt to conceal the symptom (this process is described in detail in the next chapter). They do this because it is an easy thing to do; and because this is all they know *how* to do, since their knowledge of the body's overall chemistry is still too primitive for them to be able to correct an organ's malfunctions using drugs.

There are two main problems with this approach: it does not treat the real, underlying cause, so that the person's real health issue is not addressed; and secondly, because these drugs act systemically (that is, they are everywhere in the body, through the blood stream) they also chemically block the main organs from functioning properly. And the drugs also have other random effects on the other systems in the body—hence, the wide range of adverse effects that most drugs produce, many of them unpredicted by the drug's designers.

When you stand back and consider this approach, it may seem like lunacy. But for many reasons, this approach, and also the fact that such drugs produce random, and often serious adverse effects, has become accepted. Why has it become accepted by most people that "medicine" often harms the patient? And how is such an approach even considered to be medicine? It certainly should not be, but in the collective consciousness of today's developed societies, this is an accepted reality.

The following chapters explore these issues by describing the unvarnished facts about today's pharmaceutical approach to healthcare. This includes the way drugs are designed, tested and marketed. There is also much alarming evidence of routine fraud and criminality committed by drug companies, but the purpose of this book is not to simply alarm the reader. All this evidence is necessary to demonstrate the true nature of today's mainstream healthcare system, and enables the reader to understand why it is not really healthcare at all. But the intention of this book is not to leave humanity with no healthcare. Rather, with the knowledge gained, this book aims to enable the reader to make truly informed choices about their own healthcare, and it points the way forward for a new mainstream healthcare approach.

3. The pharmaceutical approach to healthcare

Introduction

Every aspect of today's mainstream healthcare is dominated by the drug companies, which are huge commercial concerns, and, in reality, are the most unregulated industry on the planet, which will become clear in the following chapters. Their grip on mainstream healthcare is absolute. They provide all the funding; decide what should and should not be researched; which results are permitted to be made public, and which not; routinely manipulate (falsify) research data to turn negative results into positive ones, regardless of healthcare concerns; and use unscrupulous sales techniques to push knowingly inadequate products, all in the name of profit (all this is demonstrated below). Their dominance is total. Therefore, a more accurate description of today's mainstream healthcare might be "drug-company sponsored healthcare."

There are so many myths and untruths about this form of healthcare that are repeated unthinkingly by the media and medics themselves, and this has painted a general picture of a sophisticated, science-based system that does miraculous things and is a great achievement. Every aspect of this picture is untrue.

However, most people are shown this picture from early childhood, and hear it continuously from the media, so that it is not an easy task to discover the truth about mainstream healthcare.

The following sections examine each aspect as honestly as possible, providing you with the facts that drug companies would rather you did not hear, and that many medics themselves are unaware of.

What are drugs?

Most people are unaware that there is any conceptual difference between different potions and pills that are taken in response to illness. In their mind, all the different approaches are lumped into one concept. They are all simply pills taken to combat illness, and there is no conceptual difference between any of them. In this way, they do not understand the difference between a herbal potion or pill and one produced by today's drug industry.

I have even heard the comment, "Drugs are herbal remedies that have been refined to reduce the side effects." This idea is wrong on so many levels. Adverse effects are peculiar to drugs. They do not exist with herbal remedies. Also, there is no relation between most drugs and herbal remedies.

Herbs affect the body is a similar way that food does. It is often commented that food is medicine, with good reason. When one of the main organs malfunctions, this causes the person to crave a certain flavour, which happens to be the flavour that can remedy the malfunction in the organ. For example, when the pancreas function is poor, the person craves sweet tasting food; and naturally occurring sweet foods, such as root vegetables, cauliflower, rice and other grains (when all cooked) will tend to improve the pancreas function. This principle is at the root of Chinese herbal medicine, which prescribes certain natural flavours to address certain organ-related conditions.

This is perhaps how most people would understand herbs, or any medicine—simply a potion or pill that is taken to address a health issue. Therefore, they tend to imagine that today's drugs act in the same way. But this could not be more wrong.

The healing principle of herbs is abandoned by most of today's drugs, which instead are designed in response to theorizing about how the body might work, and are chemicals created to directly block the function of a healthy aspect of the body, in an attempt to stop a symptom manifesting. But because the drug acts on the entire body, it also accidentally chemically blocks the organs from being able to function normally and hence produces a wide range of unpredicted harmful effects (the adverse effects). A drug's adverse effects are, in effect, created due to man's attempts to directly take control of the body's chemistry while having an inadequate understanding of the effects of that chemis-

3. The pharmaceutical approach to healthcare

try. Hence, adverse effects only occur with today's drugs, and do not occur with properly prescribed herbal treatments.

How drugs are designed

The study of physiology has provided a basic understanding of how chemical communication within our body works. The organs release certain chemicals to control every aspect of our body. Normally, this is a complex network of activity that can change from second to second, and the communication also includes other elements that are not yet understood.[1]

But in simple terms, there are receptors (like tiny plug sockets) at various locations around our body which only accept a specific chemical (which can plug into that receptor). For example, when it is desirable to contract the muscles that surround our blood vessels, the specific chemical is released that plugs into the receptors on those muscles, and so activates the muscles. And there are very many similar actions around our body, all with their own specific receptors.

Biochemical engineers (the people who design drugs) have discovered that it is possible to design chemical agents that block certain of these receptors. And the drug companies can mass produce these chemicals, so that this crude device is now used to block the body's chemistry (to prevent certain aspects from working normally), in the hope of preventing a particular symptom from manifesting (in other words, masking the symptom).

A good example is the issue of modifying a person's blood pressure.

What is the whole "blood pressure" issue about?

When a person has high or low blood pressure, what does this mean, and why is it an issue? In all people, it is normal for our body to make constant adjustments to our blood pressure. When a stressful situation is encountered, our body responds in various ways. One of these is to adjust the muscles of our arteries and heart, so that our blood can be

Why Use Natural Healing?

circulated more rapidly, increasing the supply of nourishment which then enables us to better deal with the stressful situation. This is a perfectly normal, useful and healthy process.

If our blood pressure were measured during any stressful situation, it would be higher than when we were relaxed. This situation of temporary high blood pressure is not a disease, or even an unhealthy state; it is a perfectly normal and healthy state. It is simply a normal (and necessary) response to stress. However, in today's developed societies, it is easy for people to become locked into being constantly stressed. This is most often brought on by mental states, but physical and lifestyle factors can also cause this.

Chinese medicine fully understands how mental and emotional states are able to produce in a person the state of being constantly stressed. To treat this situation, the "meridian system" is stimulated to quickly return the person's main organs to normal function (with most patients, this would usually involve treating their liver and possibly also their "kidneys"). Once the treatment was successful, they would be more relaxed, less affected by "stressful situations", and much less likely to return to living life in a constantly stressed state. And, of course, there would not be an issue with their blood pressure, since they were no longer living life in a stressed state.

Today's mainstream healthcare, however, has no knowledge of this process of certain mental and emotional states being able to block the liver function and thus produce in us all the symptoms of stress—including constantly raised blood pressure.

What is the "pharmaceutical" thinking on this topic?

In the absence of the above knowledge, how did the current mainstream thinking on high blood pressure come about? What *is* that thinking? And how did the drug companies respond to this?

Today's study of physiology has mainly focussed on the microscopic tissue of the organs and vessels, and how the chemical communication in the body may work to control states in these structures. This physiology cannot explain and does not understand the complex interactions between our thoughts, emotions and main organ functions in the same way that Chinese medicine does. And the drug-based approach also has no way to properly return our main organs to normal function—as Chinese medicine (and other natural healing) does. Instead, because of the relatively primitive nature of the drug-based approach, the only option it has adopted is to chemically block healthy aspects of the body from working, in the hope that this will ease the patient's symptom without doing too much harm to their general health. Their approach to the blood pressure issue demonstrates this well.

How did the preoccupation with blood pressure come about?
There are great limitations in today's knowledge of physiology. These stem from the fact that it focuses on isolated tissue, and has no real knowledge of how the overall body works (when compared to the comprehensive knowledge of Chinese medicine). This means that mainstream medics are unaware of the underlying cause of most serious conditions, such as heart attacks, arterial disease, stroke, and many other serious but non-fatal conditions, such as migraines, stress-related conditions, and so on.

In the absence of this knowledge, a tool that has come to be relied on is statistical studies. When you do not know how something works, you can use statistics to make ball-park guesses.

Blood pressure is taken with most patients in mainsteam healthcare, simply because it is something that can be easily measured. When data was collected from a large number of patients who (for example) suffered heart attacks, stroke, arterial disease, and other serious conditions, it was noted that a certain percent of the patients had raised blood pressure at the culmination of their disease. Therefore it was decided, statistically, that having raised blood pressure was a possible factor that may have led to a certain number of people developing their condition.

This, of course, is not a medical fact. There is no actual knowledge of a connection between a person's blood pressure being raised, and how this might lead to a particular condition (such as heart attack, etc) developing. Instead, the statement is a statistical substitute for knowledge.

From a natural healing perspective, it is obvious that when a person is seriously ill, they are likely to be stressed, and hence will have raised blood pressure. But this does not mean that the raised blood pressure caused the illness. That notion is simply silly. However, today's physiology has no knowledge of how these conditions are caused, so they have adopted a thought pattern something like this. "If we can administer a drug that lowers the person's blood pressure, then perhaps they won't develop a serious illness. So let's do this to all people, and there's a possibility that a certain amount of them may avoid developing a serious illness where they may have otherwise."

But (as demonstrated next) the drugs that are used disable normal, healthy functions of the body, and do nothing to address any underling condition that may be there or may develop. Whatever your thoughts on this approach to medicine, it has now become the norm in mainstream healthcare, and it was this type of thinking that gave birth to the lasting preoccupation with blood pressure in mainstream healthcare.

This preoccupation has now become so prevalent that "high blood pressure" has even become labelled a "disease" in its own right, not only by many medics, but also in the public consciousness. But properly speaking, "high blood pressure" is not really a condition. It cannot even be regarded as a symptom, because it is not something the patient is even aware of. And the raising of a person's blood pressure is a normal process in a healthy person. It is not, in itself, a disease.

The drug companies being the father of today's mainstream healthcare, it was up to them to provide a solution. It is biochemical engineers who design drugs. When they consider any issue, they think about the known physiology that *could* be involved in producing that issue (in this case, blood pressure); look at the way the chemical messaging system in the body modifies this physiology; and attempt to produce drugs that block that communication, such that the physiology stops working normally, which then hides the issue. At least, that is the intention. And their hope is that the damage done to the patient's health by their intervention is kept within "acceptable" limits.

What are the common types of drugs used?

Below are listed the most common drugs, the thinking behind their design and use, the obvious flaws in this thinking, and the common adverse effects of the drugs.

Angiotensin converting enzyme (ACE) inhibitors

All the blood vessels are surrounded by a muscle layer. The purpose of this is to constantly adjust the size of the vessels, as a part of the body's management of its own blood circulation in the many different situations we find ourselves in each day (exercise of various levels, rest, sleep, or when alarmed).

To make these constant adjustments an enzyme is released into the blood, called *angiotensin converting enzyme* (ACE). This enzyme then causes the chemical *angiotensin II* to be produced in the blood, and this chemical acts on the muscles surrounding blood vessels to cause them to contract. This narrows the vessels and hence raises the blood pressure, when needed to meet our body's demands. The level of this enzyme (ACE), and hence the *angiotensin II* chemical is constantly varied by our body throughout the day to contribute to the proper functioning of our blood circulatory system, to meet our body's varying demands. This process is normal and should happen in all people for them to remain healthy.

An *ACE inhibitor* drug works by blocking the action of the ACE enzyme, which then interferes with the normal function of this regulatory mechanism, so that the blood vessels become constantly flaccid. For this reason, these drugs are sometimes known as "vasodilators". The theory is that when there is more volume in the blood (achieved by expanding the blood vessels) then by definition, there is less pressure in the blood.

Hence this drug is not correcting a health problem. In fact, it is blocking the normal function of the blood vessels.

Why Use Natural Healing?

When a person's blood pressure is constantly raised, this suggests (as mentioned on page 33) that the person has adopted mental habits that have placed them in a constantly stressed state. However, today's mainstream healthcare has no knowledge of the interaction of a person's thoughts with their main organs, and hence does not fully understand the physiology of stress. It only sees "high blood pressure" as a warning light that (in effect) must be switched off (or, more accurately "broken" to stop it flashing). And this is what the drug does. It plays a chemical trick on the body to "switch off a warning light". But mainstream healthcare does not see it this way; their thinking is that raised blood pressure is the "problem", so by applying this trick to disable this normal regulatory mechanism in the body, if this results in reduced blood pressure, they think "the problem" has been dealt with. But in fact, the underlying cause of the patient's ill health was never understood, has not been tackled, and instead an important part of the body's self regulation has been disabled.

This is only the "theoretical" effect. But because the body's overall complex chemical activity is not fully understood, when this drug is introduced, random effects occur (which the designers of the drug did not predict and are unable to explain). A good selection of these are discovered when the drug is first tried on a group of people. These are now usually called "adverse effects".[2] Some of the commonest ACE inhibitors are listed below (with trade names in brackets):

- enalapril (Vasotec)
- captopril (Capoten)
- lisinopril (Zestril and Prinivil)
- benazepril (Lotensin)
- quinapril (Accupril)
- perindopril (Aceon)
- ramipril (Altace)
- trandolapril (Mavik)
- fosinopril (Monopril)
- moexipril (Univasc)

3. The pharmaceutical approach to healthcare

Adverse effects

Some of the common adverse effects[3] of ACE inhibitors include:

- dry cough,
- loss of taste sensation,
- loss of appetite,
- shortness of breath,
- drowsiness,
- headache,
- sleep problems (insomnia),
- dry mouth,
- nausea,
- vomiting,
- diarrhoea, abdominal pain,
- skin itching or rash,
- allergic reactions with swelling of the face, lips, tongue or throat with difficulty in swallowing or breathing,
- muscle weakness,
- slow/irregular heartbeat,
- tingly feeling,
- fever,
- chills,
- persistent sore throat,
- body aches,
- flu symptoms,
- changes in the amount of urine,
- swelling, rapid weight gain,
- confusion,
- increased thirst,
- pounding heartbeats or fluttering in your chest,
- heart attack,
- fast or uneven heartbeats,
- chest pain,
- stroke,
- pale skin,
- loss of hair,
- impotence,
- easy bruising or bleeding,
- yellowing of the skin or eyes (jaundice), and
- other possible adverse effects.

This drug targets the blood-vessel muscles. But there is no claim, nor suggestion, that there is anything wrong with the blood vessel muscles, nor with the chemistry that the drug attempts to block. Therefore this intervention does not provide a "treatment". It is not curative, or healing. Instead it is purely playing a "trick" to try to hide a "warning light", without treating any aspect of the underlying problem, nor even

Why Use Natural Healing?

knowing what the underlying problem is. And with many people, this deliberate blocking of an aspect of their body's chemistry may cause them serious health problems. With several of the known adverse effects, the drug information leaflet advises you to seek emergency treatment. So, this routine remedy prescribed by mainstream healthcare could result in you requiring emergency treatment, if you are going to survive. This is a curious situation.

Angiotensin II receptor blockers (ARB's)

This drug aims to achieve the same effect as ACE inhibitors (p.37), but hopes to overcome some of the weaknesses discovered in the concept of ACE inhibitors. The blocking effect of ACE inhibitors can be bypassed in the body by other systems (reactive increase in *renin* and *angiotensin I* levels).

The ACE enzyme causes the chemical *angiotensin II* to be produced, and it is this chemical that "tells" the blood-vessel muscles to contract. And ARB's directly block the effect of the chemical *angiotensin II*, so that the blood-vessel muscles are no longer able to contract. The thinking is that even if the effects of blocking the ACE enzyme are bypassed by the body (by its complex chemistry compensating for this), the chemical that the body is still producing (*angiotensin II*) to attempt to control its blood vessels and perform other tasks, this chemical is prevented from having its effect.

Some of the commonest ARB's are listed below:
- Azilsartan (Edarbi)
- Candesartan (Atacand)
- Eprosartan
- Irbesartan (Avapro)
- Losartan (Cozaar)
- Olmesartan (Benicar)
- Telmisartan (Micardis)
- Valsartan (Diovan)

It is said that these drugs have less adverse effects than ACE inhibitors, though the known adverse effects can still be serious, and all the same comments apply. As before, there is no claim that there is anything wrong with the body's chemistry that this drug attempts to block and it is therefore not providing a "treatment" (it is not healing or curative) but is merely attempting to switch off a warning light and hence mask the real underlying problem; and in the process, it may seriously harm your health.

Beta-blockers

When we need to perform better, or more quickly (which is usually the case in most stressful situations), our main organs (primarily the "kidneys", which include the adrenal glands) release the hormones adrenaline and noradrenaline. Many of the organs, systems and vessels in the body have receptors on them that detect this hormone in the blood; when detected, they adjust their behaviour, so as to enable us to respond to the stressful situation. These receptors are called *adrenergic beta receptors*. The beta-blocker drug prevents these receptors from detecting the adrenaline hormone. One of the effects of this is to slow our heart rate, which can then lead to lowered blood pressure.

There are three known types of beta receptors, and some beta-blockers are able to target one particular type of beta receptor. The receptors are located in the heart, kidneys, lungs, gut, liver, uterus, blood vessels, fat cells, and in the skeletal muscles. Hence, our main organs would usually attempt to adjust many aspects of our body to respond to stressful situations. This is normal, and essential for our immediate and long-term survival.

Beta-blockers can impede any part, or even the whole, of this system. As usual, the drug is not given to a patient to "treat" a condition, in that there is usually nothing wrong with this entire "fight-or-flight system" (as it is usually called). Therefore, the drug has no "medical" intention, or healing effect. Instead, this fight-or-flight system is being chemically impeded simply to attempt to switch off the "high-blood-pressure warning light", usually with no knowledge of the genuine, underlying condition (the reason why the person is now locked into living in a constantly stressed state, and hence having raised blood pressure).

This fight-or-flight system is present in many key organs and systems of our body, and our main organs normally regulate it throughout the day, making continuous fine adjustments. As can be imagined, any interference with this chemistry could produce a wide range of adverse effects, some serious or even fatal.

Adverse effects

Currently known adverse affects of beta blockers include:

- nausea,
- diarrhoea,
- bronchospasm (causing difficulty in breathing, possibly severe),
- shortness of breath,
- cold extremities,
- slow heart beat,
- heart failure,
- disruption of the heart's electrical impulses,
- fatigue,
- dizziness,
- hair loss,
- abnormal vision,
- hallucinations,
- insomnia,
- nightmares,
- sexual dysfunction,
- type 2 diabetes, and
- other possible adverse effects.

Calcium channel blockers (CCBs)

Calcium channels are pores in cells that allow calcium to pass into the cell. A calcium element is known as an ion. This is because it has an unequal number of protons and electrons, which gives it a positive charge of 2. When ions exist in liquid form (as calcium does within our body), this provides a way for the body to move electrical charge around. When a calcium ion enters a cell through its calcium channel, this increases the electrical charge on that cell, and the cell then uses this charge for various purposes. This process is used by nerves to produce an electrical impulse, and it also plays a key role in the function of smooth muscle, enabling it to contract.

Our blood vessels are surrounded by smooth muscle. But when these calcium channels are blocked, this prevents the muscle from working, so that the muscle loses its normal control and becomes flaccid.

This "trick" is used to cause the blood vessels to unnaturally expand, and from a pure plumbing point of view, because there is now more volume for the blood to fill, this means that the pressure of the blood is reduced. In the same way, if you expanded the pipes in your home's plumbing system, the water pressure would be reduced.

As before, there is no suggestion that there is any fault in this mechanism. Therefore, this drug does not have a healing effect. It is not directly correcting a problem. But rather, it is preventing a normal and vital system in the body from working properly, so as to hide a warning light about something somewhere else in the body; and leaving that underlying condition in place. So, as usual, not only does this type of approach, not do any good for the body, or provide any cure, but it actively prevents a separate part of the body (or a whole system) from working, a part or system that was previously working perfectly.

Smooth muscle exists in many parts of the body. One important location is within the lymphatic system; and when this smooth muscle is prevented from working properly, the normal lymph drainage in the body fails to work, causing swelling of tissue.

This is an obvious adverse effect; this is so obvious, the drug designers are able to predict and expect it. But (as with most drugs) many other adverse effects were not predicted, and it is not known how the symptoms are produced. This is only to be expected when the body's complex chemistry is impeded in any way.

Adverse effects

Common adverse effects[4] of calcium channel blockers include:

- headache,
- constipation,
- rash,
- nausea,
- flushing,
- edema (fluid accumulation in tissues),
- drowsiness,
- low blood pressure,
- dizziness

Why Use Natural Healing?

- sexual dysfunction,
- overgrowth of gums,
- liver dysfunction,
- some CCB's may worsen heart failure, and
- other possible adverse effects.

Diuretics

One aspect of the normal kidney function is to filter blood to remove harmful or unneeded elements from the blood, and then to reabsorb the "cleansed" water back into the blood, to help maintain the body's necessary liquid levels.

There are several different types of diuretic drug. They all aim to block this normal process of reabsorbing "clean" water back into the blood, but each type of drug achieves this by disabling a different aspect of the kidneys. The intention here is that, from a pure plumbing point of view, if there is less water in the blood, then there is less volume in the "pipes" (the blood vessels), therefore, the pressure in the pipes will be less (the blood pressure is lower).

Again, there is no suggestion that there is anything wrong with your kidneys in the first place, so the chemical blocking of your normal kidney function is not producing a healing effect, and is not even intended to "correct" a problem with your kidneys in any way. Instead (as usual), the chemical blocking of your normal kidney function is being done to hide a warning light about some other underlying problem, but without addressing that problem, and not usually even knowing what that problem is.

Adverse effects

There are many obvious and predicted adverse effects[5] when the tissues of your body are robbed of the essential water they need. These, and other adverse effects, are:

- dry mouth,
- thirst,
- weakness,
- lethargy,

- drowsiness,
- restlessness,
- muscle pains or cramps,
- confusion,
- seizures,
- muscular fatigue,
- hypotension,
- oliguria (decreased or absent production of urine),
- increased heartbeat,
- gastrointestinal disturbances,
- death (caused by extremely low levels of sodium),
- neurologic damage,
- gout (from increased uric acid levels),
- other possible adverse effects.

Alpha-blockers

This chemical is another approach used to attempt to prevent the smooth muscle that surrounds blood vessels from working properly.

Alpha-blockers work by blocking the transmission of certain nerve impulses. When some nerves are stimulated, they release a chemical called *noradrenaline* into the blood. This chemical then stimulates *alpha-adrenergic* receptors, which exist in various parts of the body, including the heart, smooth muscle and blood vessels. When these receptors are stimulated, they cause blood vessels to constrict. This is an essential process that the body uses to maintain the normal function of the heart and blood vessels under varying conditions.

An alpha-blocker drug attaches to these *alpha-adrenergic* receptors and blocks them from being stimulated. This action prevents the smooth muscle that surrounds blood vessels from working, and the blood vessels become flaccid.

Again, when this drug is used, there is no suggestion that there is any fault with this system, so the drug is not providing any healing effect in the body. Instead it is disabling this healthy tissue from working properly, so as to hide a warning light that some unknown thing is wrong elsewhere.

Common alpha-blockers include:
- Alfuzosin (Uroxatral)

Why Use Natural Healing?

- Doxazosin (Cardura)
- Prazosin (Minipress)
- Silodosin (Rapaflo)
- Tamsulosin (Flomax)
- Terazosin (Hytrin)

Adverse effects

Common adverse effects[6] of alpha-blockers include:
- dizziness, sometimes severe
- lightheadedness,
- headache,
- fatigue,
- tired feeling,
- stuffy nose, sneezing, or sore throat,
- fainting,
- fast or irregular heartbeat, or
- chest pain.

Adverse effects not usually mentioned

With all drugs, the total list of known adverse effects is always much longer than the list usually mentioned to patients by medics or informational websites. This is partly because the list, if given for *all* patients, could be literally endless. Different people respond in different ways to the same drug, and some people are more sensitive than others. Also, many of the effects are not known by drug companies, because they may take years to build up and medics may never associate the adverse affect with the drug that caused it. They simply consider it to be a separate, unrelated symptom.

However, looking at the patient information leaflet for any drug, should report a full list of the adverse effects noticed when the drug was first tried on patients, or reported to the drug company later. This full list is always much longer than the common effects usually mentioned.

For example, with the above drug (alfuzosin, or Uroxatral), the list of common adverse effects usually mentioned only includes 9 items,

3. The pharmaceutical approach to healthcare

but the complete list in the patient information leaflet includes 32 items, some serious:

- feeling dizzy or faint,
- headache,
- feeling sick,
- weakness or tiredness,
- diarrhoea,
- stomach pain,
- general feeling of being unwell,
- feeling dizzy, light-headed or faint when you stand,
- dry mouth,
- being sick (vomiting),
- a fast heart beat (tachycardia),
- pounding in the chest and uneven heartbeat (palpitations),
- chest pain,
- drowsiness,
- rash and itching,
- hot flushes,
- problems with your vision,
- runny nose, itching, sneezing, stuffy nose and/or burning eyes,
- water retention (may cause swollen arms or legs),
- lack of control over passing water,
- fainting,
- uncomfortable feeling in the stomach and indigestion (dyspepsia),
- abnormal liver function (signs may include yellowing of your skin or the whites of your eyes),
- you may get more infections than usual,
- abnormal heart rhythm,
- impaired brain function,
- increased risk of bleeding (including nose bleeds and/or bleeding gums) and bruising,

- swelling of the hands, feet, ankles, face, lips or throat which may cause difficulty in swallowing or breathing,
- itchy, lumpy rash (hives) or nettle rash (urticaria),
- chest pain (angina),
- painful erection of the penis, not related to sexual activity, which will not go away.

Alpha-beta blockers

These drugs are intended to have the effect of both beta-blockers (p.41) and alpha-blockers (p.45). The arguments in those sections also apply to alpha-beta blockers.

Other drugs

Drugs of other types may also be tried to address the "high blood pressure" issue. These could include drugs such as clonidine, aliskiren (Tekturna), and minoxidil. They have similar effects to the drugs mentioned above, but act by blocking other aspects of the body's chemistry.

With all the above drugs, what should be remembered is that "high blood pressure" by itself is not a condition; and the chemistry that these drugs block in your body is not faulty in any way; there is nothing wrong with it. And blocking that chemistry, only causes further problems. Instead "high blood pressure" is at best a warning light that something else is not right. But because the focus of mainstream healthcare has been guided by drug companies for so long, this has precluded it from even being able to detect the real underlying condition.

To understand why this is so, it is necessary to understand what natural healing is, and how it diagnoses a problem and successfully heals it. Only by understanding this, it is possible to see today's mainstream approach to healthcare in context, and therefore gain the insights that would enable you to make a genuinely informed choice about your healthcare.

4. How does natural healing treat "blood pressure" issues?

In Chinese medicine, a patient's blood pressure is not normally taken. In my own acupuncture practice, I only take a patient's blood pressure when they are taking drugs prescribed for that issue and they wish to come off the drugs. I take their blood pressure through the course of treatments, purely for the patient's peace of mind. And I find that the more they reduce such drugs, the more their blood pressure returns to normal. Admittedly this is while they are receiving acupuncture treatment, and it could be said that the withdrawal of such drugs allows the acupuncture treatment to have its full effect, which is the explanation for their blood pressure returning to normal.

Note that such drugs tend to block natural healing from working. In natural healing, it is the organs themselves that do the healing, by returning to normal function; but when a patient takes such drugs, their organs cannot adjust their own functions because the body's chemistry (which is one of their main means of communication) is blocked.

In other circumstances, we never take a patient's blood pressure. Instead, there are many diagnostic methods used, which are powerful and have stood the test of time.

When someone has consistently high blood pressure, what is happening physiologically in their body? The body increases blood pressure whenever a stressful situation is encountered. It is an emergency measure, to enable us to cope with that emergency. When a person's blood pressure remains high continuously, this implies that their main organs have been "tricked" into thinking the body is under constant stress.

Chinese medicine knowledge of the interaction between our thoughts and main organs, suggests that the organs involved are probably the liver and "kidneys", and sometimes poor function of the lungs may also be involved.

Why Use Natural Healing?

When we say "kidneys" in Chinese medicine, this includes three structures: the kidneys, adrenal glands and sex organs, all treated as a single organ. The adrenal glands are universally recognised as being a key organ in our response to stressful situations (in the release of adrenaline). And Chinese medicine knowledge recognises that stagnated liver function produces most of the physical and mental symptoms related to stress.

It is also recognised that poor "kidney" function, and sometimes also poor lung function, tend to cause the liver function to stagnate.

The complex and ever-changing communication between these organs and our body is not understood. The communication uses a combination of chemical, hormonal and nervous signals; and possibly other methods of communication (which are only recently beginning to be explored[1]), which may involve organ information conveyed around the body (and beyond) on electromagnetic waves, which travel around 670 times faster than nerve impulses travel.[2]

This complex communication between the organs is not understood, which is one good reason why it is not advisable to attempt to block any aspect of the body's chemistry. However, Chinese medicine knows nothing about this communication, and does not *need* to understand it, and, of course, never tries to manipulate it or take control of it.

How is an accurate diagnosis made?

There is a wide range of techniques that a Chinese medicine practitioner uses to make a diagnosis. As mentioned starting on page 14, this could include tongue examination; feeling the organ "pulses"; pressing key "acupoints" on an organ's meridian; questioning the patient about their symptoms; and observing their behaviour. Each of these indicators alone can usually tell the practitioner which organs need treating, but it is usual for the practitioner to use several of these techniques to confirm the diagnosis. All this knowledge was amassed over thousands of years of clinical experience, and has been stable over all that time.

The association between each organ and the range of symptoms that occur when that organ is not functioning well (pages 9 to 13), was first worked out over 2,000 years ago in ancient China; and I am often amazed at just how accurate these associations are today. Sometimes when taking a case history from a new patient, it can seem as though the patient has read a Chinese medicine textbook and is simply reciting the list of symptoms associated with a particular organ. Of course they have not read such a book, and are just relaying the symptoms they have noticed in themselves. But the accuracy of these associations (2,000 years later) is often uncanny.

The sensitivity of Chinese medicine

However, today's approach to healthcare is blind to this entire body of knowledge. Usually, when a person is ill, and the reason for their symptoms is obvious to a traditional acupuncture practitioner, today's medics are often unable to detect an organ-related problem that could explain the symptom. For this reason, it is clear that this range of diagnostic techniques makes Chinese medicine far more sensitive than today's mainstream healthcare.

Not only does today's mainstream healthcare not possess this knowledge of the physical and mental symptoms associated with each organ, but also, the medics have no training in how to use their own senses and ability to detect problems in the organ functions. The devices and blood tests available to them are also unable to detect these organ malfunctions that produce most common symptoms. This only reduces the sensitivity of mainstream healthcare. But another big problem is that, even if medics were told which organ functions needed correcting, they would have no way of returning those organs to normal function. The drug industry has mainly learnt how to block the chemistry of the body (in the pursuit of misguided goals); or, in the absence of being able to heal, to wage war on pathogens (Chapter 10). And there is no way that blocking any element of the body's chemistry would be able to correct organ malfunctions—since the organs need to be able to control that chemistry themselves to function normally; and also any such drugs risk directly blocking the very fabric of the organs from working, which would also prevent them from functioning normally.

Once discovered, how are faults in the organ functions treated?
When any organ malfunctions, including the liver, kidneys or lungs (the organs that are most likely to affect blood pressure), each organ's state is reflected at various locations along its related meridian. This happens because of a resonance that has formed throughout evolution between each organ and certain locations on the body. These locations are called acupuncture points (or acupoints). When the related organ functions poorly, the tissue at its main acupoints also functions poorly. This means that when that acupoint is pressed by your practitioner, it would feel tender to you, as though it had been bruised; that is, as though the local tissue had been damaged. This "damaged" state is simply a reflection of the "damaged" state of the related organ's tissue while that organ is not functioning normally.

When one of these tender acupoints is stimulated, this same resonance between the acupoint and its related organ, works in reverse. The stimulation tends to cause the local tissue to return to normal function (and it is no longer tender when pressed; is no longer acting as though bruised), and because of the resonance between this acupoint and the related organ, the organ is also prompted to return to normal function.

This transformation usually happens in a few seconds. At this point, all the diagnostic indicators would indicate that the organ function was now normal. This would be apparent in the organ "pulses"; on the patient's tongue; in the fact that all the organ's key acupoints would no longer feel tender when pressed (even if they had not been needled); many types of anomaly, such as redness or coldness, would no longer be present on the skin along the organ's related meridian; and the patient would feel greatly relaxed, due to the absence of the stressed state within their organs that they were used to feeling. Any of these diagnostic techniques can be tested to confirm that the organ concerned was now functioning normally.

This treatment of the organs was achieved by the practitioner taking part in a subtle way in the "conversation" between those organs and the patient's body. That is, the natural "conversation" of the organs was "nudged" to return the entire organ system to normal function. Nothing foreign to the body, or foreign to each organ's regulatory mecha-

4. How does natural healing treat "blood pressure" issues?

nisms, was introduced. The organs themselves performed the healing, using all their own normal devices. This means, of course, that any adjustment that occurred in the body's complex and ever-changing chemistry was performed by the organs themselves. This is as it should be, since it is only the organ's themselves that understand this complex "conversation". Humanity certainly does not understand it.

The approach of mainstream healthcare

As mentioned before, "high blood pressure" is not a real condition, nor even a symptom, since the patient is not usually aware of it (pages 33-37). It is simply a measurement that today's mainstream healthcare can easily perform. But that healthcare system does not understand the real underlying condition, so it has come to regard this measurement (high blood pressure) as a disease in its own right. In effect, it has invented this "disease".

Once a "condition" has been identified (whether real or not), how does mainstream healthcare tackle this?

The approach was clearly portrayed in the sections on common drugs used in response to the "high blood pressure" issue (pages 37 to 48), where it was shown that the approach was, in effect, to attempt to block the chemistry of a normally functioning system in the body, with the aim of "switching off a warning light" that indicated something was wrong elsewhere in the body. To fully demonstrate the effect on the patient of this approach, I will look at a single drug and use the insights from Chinese medicine to work out which organ functions may be accidentally affected by the drug.

The following passage analyses the drug *lisinopril* (brand names: Prinivil, or Zestril), which is currently the most commonly prescribed drug for high blood pressure.[3] Though I am focusing on *lisinopril*, all the same principles and comments apply to most of the commonly used drugs, including those for other "conditions".

What type of drug is this?
This drug is known as an ACE inhibitor. See page 37 for a description of the body's chemistry that this drug seeks to block.

Why Use Natural Healing?

What are the possible adverse effects of taking this drug?
Advice to patients published on websites and elsewhere, usually lists around eight common adverse effects, including:

- dizziness,
- cough,
- headache,
- high potassium levels,
- diarrhoea,
- low blood pressure,
- chest pain, and
- fatigue.

Using Chinese medicine knowledge of the symptoms produced when each organ's function is disrupted (pages 9 to 13), it is clear that this drug impedes the lung function (producing a persistent dry cough), the pancreas function (producing diarrhoea and fatigue), possibly also the "kidney" function (contributing to fatigue), and possibly the heart function (producing chest pain).

From the physiology point of view, it is unclear how blocking the particular chemistry in the body that this drug does, could produce a cough, diarrhoea or fatigue. The other adverse effects above could possibly be explained by the action of disabling the function of the smooth muscle in the blood vessels and elsewhere in the body.

However this type of "physiology" explanation is largely guesswork. Current physiology does not fully understand the complex communication that takes place between the systems in the body (and is not even aware of some aspects of this communicatoin—p.50), therefore when one element of this complex network is blocked, the results may appear to be random.

This is made clear by the much larger list of recorded adverse effects that appear in only selected people. The apparent randomness of this pattern, and the inexplicable nature of some of the adverse effects demonstrates that the current knowledge of the chemical communication in the body is inadequate. This is why it is not possible to predict the adverse effects that may occur when any patient first takes this drug (and most other drugs).

In the patient information leaflet, a more comprehensive list of adverse effects is published. This list includes all the adverse affects that were noticed among the large group of patients whom the drug was first tried on. Therefore, these adverse effects are not theoretical; these are the effects that occurred in reality when the drug was given to patients.

In the following list of symptoms, if Chinese medicine knowledge can identify which organ was affected by the drug to produce that particular symptom, the organ is mentioned in brackets.

1 in 10 people experienced:
- headache
- feeling dizzy or light-headed (**liver or "kidneys"**)
- diarrhoea (**pancreas**)
- dry cough that does not go away (**lungs**)
- vomiting (**stomach**)
- kidney problems (**kidneys**)

1 in 100 people experienced:
- mood changes (**liver**)
- change of colour in your fingers or toes (pale blue followed by redness) or numbness or tingling in your fingers or toes
- changes in the way things taste (**pancreas**)
- feeling sleepy (**pancreas or "kidneys"**)
- spinning feeling (**liver or "kidneys"**)
- having difficulty sleeping (**heart**)
- stroke (**"kidneys"**)
- fast heart beat (**heart**)
- inflammation of the nose lining, characterized by a blocked or runny nose and sneezing (**lungs**)
- feeling sick (**stomach, or liver**)
- stomach pain or indigestion (**stomach**)
- skin rash or itching

Why Use Natural Healing?

- being unable to get an erection (**"kidneys"**)
- feeling tired or feeling weak (**pancreas**)
- heart attack (**heart**)
- seen and/or heard hallucinations

1 to 1,000 people experienced:
- feeling confused
- lumpy rash
- dry mouth
- hair loss (**"kidneys"**)
- psoriasis
- changes in the way things smell (**lungs**)
- development of breasts in men (**"kidneys"**)
- blood disorders; e.g. a drop in blood haemoglobin levels, reduction in haematocrit
- changes to some of the cells or other parts of your blood, which may produce symptoms of: feeling tired, pale skin, a sore throat, fever, joint and muscle pains, swelling of the joints or glands, or sensitivity to sunlight
- sudden renal failure (**kidneys**)
- mental confusion (possibly **"kidneys" or heart**)
- severe allergic reactions, producing: swelling of your face, lips, tongue or throat; difficult to swallow; severe or sudden swelling of your hands, feet and ankles; difficulty breathing; severe itching of the skin with raised lumps
- a sudden build-up of fluid in the skin, throat and tongue, breathing difficulties and/or itching and skin rash, often as an allergic reaction

1 in 10,000 people experienced:
- tight-chestedness, pain and fullness behind your cheeks and eyes, pneumonia (**lungs**)
- wheezing (**lungs**)

- low levels of sugar in your blood, feeling hungry or weak, sweating, dizziness and a fast heart beat (**pancreas, "kidneys"**)
- inflammation of the liver, leading to loss of appetite, yellowing of the skin and eyes, and a dark coloured urine (**liver**)
- inflammation of the pancreas, causing moderate to severe pain in the upper stomach radiating to the back, as well as nausea and vomiting, abdominal pain, inflammation of the liver accompanied by jaundice (**pancreas and liver**)
- blood and lymphatic system disorders accompanied by an increased susceptibility to infections, anaemia, haemolytic anaemia (**lymphatic system**)
- sweating
- passing less urine than normal or passing no water (**kidneys**)
- liver failure (**liver**)
- lumps
- inflamed gut (**pancreas**)
- severe skin disorders, like a sudden, unexpected rash or burning, red or peeling skin
- an infection with symptoms such as fever and serious deterioration of your general condition, or fever with local infection symptoms such as sore throat/pharynx/mouth or urinary problems
- serious blood disorder (a lack of white blood cells) accompanied by an increased susceptibility to infections, or by sudden high fever, severe sore throat and mouth ulcers

An unknown number of people experienced:
- symptoms of depression (**liver**)
- fainting
- inflamed blood vessels
- muscle pain
- painful joints
- inflamed joints
- hypersensitivity to sunlight and other skin reactions.

The frequency of a particular adverse effect (1 in 10, or 1 in 100, etc), is irrelevant. This simply reflects the fact that people are complex, and each person responds differently (or at a different speed) to the same drug. This unpredictability and apparent randomness, simply confirms that drug designers (biochemical engineers) do not have the ability to predict what will happen when the body's complex chemistry is impeded with a drug.

Analysis of all the currently known adverse effects

From the above lists of known adverse effects, Chinese medicine knowledge suggests that the organs adversely affected (mentioned in brackets) include the pancreas, lungs, kidneys (and adrenal glands and gonads), stomach, heart, liver, and the lymphatic system.

These drugs impede the function of all our important organs

With the above drug, the intention of the drug designer was to try to block the function of one aspect of the patient's body, such as the muscular layer surrounding their blood vessels. But instead, it is clear that the drug blocks the function of all the patient's main organs (as demonstrated above).* Because the drug is systemic (reaches every part of the body, through the blood supply) this effect is not surprising.

In summary, such drugs are prescribed to attempt to correct a condition that is, in effect, fictitious. The doctor is unaware of the real underlying problem, and the drug deliberately blocks a healthy function in the body and in doing this it accidentally harms the patient's health.

Such an approach to healthcare is, of course, extremely reckless. And why on earth (you might ask) would any developed civilization allow this approach to be used?

---

* The speed and degree of this effect would vary from person to person, but if the drug were taken long term, it would be surprising if the effect was not seriously detrimental to most patient's long-term health.

4. How does natural healing treat "blood pressure" issues?

Most people, including most medics, are unaware of the true nature of drug remedies and how they affect the body. This is because the publicity and sales arms of the drug industry have concocted an array of nifty phrases that make this whole approach seem normal, acceptable, and even desirable (Chapter 13). This is a sinister mirage, but these phrases now trip off the tongues of doctors, the media, and the majority of unsuspecting citizens. But to be able to properly understand this topic, you need to know the truth about how drug companies operate, which is described in the following chapters.

5. The conduct of drug companies

To understand how harmful the pharmaceutical industry has become to global healthcare, and how much of an illusion the industry has created around its activities, it is necessary to understand the way they conduct themselves when designing and marketing drugs, and the nature of their influence in all mainstream healthcare matters.

The main message of this chapter is not that common drugs are harmful and even lethal. They are both of these things. For example

- in the USA it has been reported that every year around 200,000 people die from adverse reactions from prescribed drugs;[1, 2, 3]
- a Norwegian study found that 18% of people who die in hospital, die because of the drugs they were given in hospital;[4] and
- the EU has estimated that adverse drug reactions also kill around 200,000 people every year in Europe.[5]

These figures demonstrate that in the United States and Europe, adverse reactions to prescription drugs are the third leading cause of death, after heart disease and cancer. However, the actual figures are probably much higher, as many deaths from drug reactions are impossible to trace. For example, many drugs cause heart failure, which would usually be recorded as death from natural causes. And in addition to these deaths, millions of people suffer serious, disabling drug injuries every year.[6]

These facts should not be too much of a surprise (strangely, that drugs have adverse reactions has become an accepted part of mainstream healthcare). Instead, the main message of this chapter is the dishonesty of drug companies in deliberately concealing the known harms of their key products (by, for example, concealing the deaths that occur when they trial a drug); and in extensively manipulating trial data to create the fraudulent illusion that their drug remedies are effective (while knowing that they have no beneficial effect, and only harm patients). These facts are demonstrated in the following chapters. The interesting question this raises is, "Why do drug companies need to be so dishonest?" If they had a product that worked, there would be no need for their dishonestly.

Serious harms concealed, purely for profit

This section gives many examples of major drug companies deliberately concealing serious harms caused by their drugs.

Thalidomide

In 1957, the German company Grünenthal, first marketed their drug thalidomide. They promoted it for morning sickness (amongst other things), though it hadn't been adequately tested in pregnant animals.[7] Before long, Grünenthal started receiving reports of children being born without arms or legs, which they ignored. Then a German physician found 14 cases of rare birth defects related to the drug, and reported these to them. The company already knew about the birth defects and also had about 2,000 reports of serious irreversible nerve damage caused by the drug. However, they kept these reports secret, and responded to the doctor by threatening legal action. They also sent 70,000 letters to other German doctors stating that thalidomide was a safe drug, and they hired private detectives to monitor any physicians who criticized the drug.[7] Grünenthal harassed the doctor for the next ten years. They also harassed and intimidated an FDA scientist who refused to approve thalidomide for the US market.

Astra, Scandinavia's biggest drug company, manufactured thalidomide. In 1965, the first court cases against them began. But lawyers had enormous difficulty finding experts who were willing to testify against Astra.[7] And in the USA, the company that distributed thalidomide (even though it was not approved by the FDA) hired every expert there was on birth defects to prevent them from testifying for the victims. In the German court cases, the drug company's defence was to argue that it wasn't against the law to damage a foetus, as it had no legal rights. Eventually, the trial ended with a meagre settlement of around $11,000 for each deformed baby.

In the UK, journalists were not permitted to write about the UK court cases. The *Sunday Times* had described incriminating evidence against the drug, but publication was blocked by the UK government (under Margaret Thatcher), who were more concerned about protecting the profits of the drug companies. After ten years, the cases ended up in the EU courts, who were baffled by the UK government's stance. The European Commission issued a report that contained the censored *Sunday Times* article, which had now eventually been made public after sixteen years.

Antidepressant-related suicides concealed by drug companies

A group of drugs known as *selective serotonin reuptake inhibiter* (SSRI) are used as antidepressants. They are designed to increase the levels of serotonin in the brain, and hence make people feel happier. Common examples are: fluoxetine (Prozac or Oxactin) and paroxetine (Paxil, Seroxat).

In 2001, GlaxoSmithKline published a trial of their drug Paxil, conducted on children and adolescents diagnosed with depression (which became known as study 329).[8] The study concluded that the drug was "generally well tolerated and effective for major depression in adolescents". But in 2004, New York State sued the company for repeated and persistent consumer fraud in relation to concealing harms of Paxil,[9] and the company's archives were disclosed as a part of the settlement. This revealed internal company documents which acknowledged that study 329 did not show that Paxil was effective. It was negative for effectiveness and positive for harm. It was also revealed that a PR firm had been used to ghost write the study, and that the data was extensively manipulated to hide the serious harms and produce the false claims of effectiveness. The genuine data (only revealed through litigation) showed that at least eight children became suicidal on Paxil, and only one on placebo; and there were also eleven serious adverse effects amongst the 93 children treated with Paxil. This indicated that the harmfulness of Paxil was serious and statistically significant. Internal documents also revealed that the company lied to its sales force that Paxil showed "Remarkable efficacy and safety."

The drug industry employs well-practiced tricks to manipulate trial data in a drug's favour. In study 329, five case of suicidal thoughts and behaviour in the children taking Paxil, were instead recorded as "emotional lability", and three extra cases of suicidal thoughts or self-harm were listed as "hospitalization". Also, at least three adolescents receiving Paxil in the trial, threatened or attempted suicide; but the report's main author, Martin Keller, stated that they were terminated from the study due to "non-compliance".[9]

Another "non-compliant" teenager took 82 tablets of paracetamol (a lethal dose), and it appears he was removed from the study, and instead a new teenager took his place (being assigned the same number). This raises the possibility that other teenagers who suffered serious harm in the trial were simply removed from the trial, to conceal the damning evidence. When the FDA asked the company to review the study data again, the company now "found" four additional cases of self-injury, suicidal ideas or suicidal attempts, all while taking Paxil.

At the time, it was the custom for drug companies to pay doctors $25,000 for each vulnerable teenager they could enrol into a drug trial. And a list of such teenagers has been discovered, as though having been entered for a trial, but no trial was being conducted. Massachusetts Department of Mental Health is reported to have also paid the psychiatric depart that Martin Keller (the lead author of study 329) chaired, hundreds of thousands of dollars to fund research that was not even being conducted.[9]

Glaxo was aware that Paxil did not work for children and was seriously harmful for them (which the company had concealed), but despite this, Glaxo heavily promoted the drug for use in children. And the drug was not even approved for use in children. The company was charged with illegal marketing, which involved withholding trials showing Paxil was ineffective.[10]

However, it is not difficult to see Glaxo's motivating factor. Between 1998 and 2001, 15 million prescriptions were written for Paxil and Zoloft (a Pfizer SSRI) for children and adolescents, in the USA alone.[11] With such colossal sales, any litigation or fines for fraud or damages must seem a minor inconvenience.

Apart from other adverse effects, such drugs clearly affect a person's mind. Peter Gøtzsche's 2017 book[12] provides many harrowing accounts of otherwise healthy people being prescribed SSRI's and then succumbing to suicide, sometimes after murdering family members, and often after suffering other disturbing adverse effects for weeks.

An industry-wide practice
David Healy performed a study of sertraline (a Pfizer SSRI) in 20 healthy volunteers with no history of depression or mental illness. On taking the drug, 2 of them became suicidal, and both remained disturbed for several months and seriously questioned the stability of their personalities.[13] Pfizer's own studies in healthy volunteers showed similar adverse effects, but this data remained hidden in company files.[13]

Reviewers at the US Food and Drug Administration (FDA) found that the big drug companies had concealed cases of suicidal thoughts and acts by labelling them "emotional lability".[13, 14, 15] But the FDA suppressed this information. And when safety officer Andrew Mosholder concluded that SSRI's caused increased suicidality among teenagers, the FDA also suppressed his report. When the report was leaked, the FDA's only response was to launch a criminal investigation into the leak,[15, 16] confirming that their allegiances lay with drug companies, not the public.

Data uncovered from the FDA by David Healy[17] showed drug company manipulation of trial data to hide serious adverse effects. In a sertraline trail[18] there had been five suicidal attempts by the participants while under the influence of the drug, but the company had fraudulently recorded three of the attempts as occurring in the placebo group (who did not receive the drug), thus making the drug seem statistically safe, compared to the placebo group. These facts were not denied by either Pfizer[19] or Glaxo.[20]

At least three companies, Glaxo, Lilly and Pfizer, concealed suicides that occurred during trials of their drugs, by manipulating the trial data in this same way—fraudulently moving the suicidal participants to the placebo group to create the statistical illusion that their drug did not induce suicidal thoughts.[13, 17, 21, 22, 23]

Apart from enabling them to successfully market harmful drugs, this device also provides them with a degree of legal protection when their drugs cause harm. A man taking paroxetine (a Glaxo SSRI) murdered his wife, daughter and granddaughter and committed suicide, but in its defence Glaxo stated that its published trials of the drug did not show an increased risk of suicide.[23]

In 2004, a systematic review of SSRI trials showed that when unpublished trials were included, the risk versus benefit factor for taking the drug was transformed from favourable to unfavourable for several of the SSRIs.[24] In other words, the drug companies did not publish any trials that demonstrated the harm of their drugs, and only published the trials where they had manipulated the data to give a false favourable impression for their drug.

In 2004, Toshi Furukawa used the full reports of Glaxo's trials (which were made available on the internet as a result of litigation), and found that paroxetine now increased significantly suicidal tendencies.[14] In other words, Glaxo had kept secret, trial data that showed their drug induced suicidal tendencies, so as to give the opposite impression in the trials that they did publish. He included three unpublished trials. One of these was "study 377" which showed that paroxetine was no better than placebo (in other words, it showed that the drug did not work—see p.79). In an internal document,[25] Glaxo had stated that "There are no plans to publish data from Study 377." He also included study 329, which he found had manipulated the trial data to hide the harmful effects of the trial drug. Self harm and suicidal thoughts had been hidden in the results by calling them something else. An 11 year-old boy threatened to harm himself and was hospitalized; this was described in the data as "exacerbated depression". And a 14 year-old boy had harmed himself, expressed hopelessness and possible suicidal thoughts and was hospitalized; this was described in the trial data as a case of "aggression".

Ciba (Novartis) covers up paralysis caused by its diarrhoea drug

In 1934, a Swiss company, Ciba (now Novartis), launched a drug for diarrhoea, called clioquinol. By 1953, Ciba was marketing the drug worldwide for all types of dysentery. But the drug was neurotoxic and caused a disaster in Japan, where (by 1972) 10,000 people had developed symptoms of tingling in the feet that eventually turned into total loss of sensation and then paralysis of the feet and legs. Others suffered blindness and other serious eye disorders. Ciba knew about the harms but concealed them for many years.[26] When the Japanese disaster became known, Ciba lied that their drug could not be responsible because it was insoluble and could not be absorbed by the body (despite the company knowing that it could be absorbed).[27] In 1965, a Swiss vet found that dogs treated with clioquinol developed acute epileptic convulsions and died. Ciba's response was merely to insert a warning in the drug's packaging in England that it should not be used in animals. In 1966, two Swedish paediatricians found that a 3-year-old boy treated with clioquinol had suffered severely impaired vision. They reported their findings and also informed Ciba that clioquinol was absorbed and could damage the optic nerve. Despite these events, including the Japanese disaster, the company continued marketing the drug worldwide. By 1976, the drug was still available over-the-counter for travellers' diarrhoea, despite the harms and the lack of evidence that it was effective.[28] By 1981, Ciba-Geigy had paid out over $490 million to Japanese victims, but the company did not take the drug off the market until 1985, 15 years after the Japanese disaster began.

Asthma inhaler-deaths covered up by drug companies

In the 1960's, inhalers for asthma were first marketed. Deaths from asthma then rose sharply, in parallel with the sales of these drugs. Regulators warned about overuse, and the drug sales declined, matched by a reduction in deaths. Neil Pearce, from New Zealand, studied one of these drugs, *isoprenaline*. His study confirmed the theory that these drugs had been responsible for the deaths, but the drug company, Riker, rigorously denied this, threatening him with litigation.[29] In 1976 a new epidemic of asthma deaths began in New Zealand. Pearce and his colleagues discovered that the new epidemic also mirrored the sales for an inhaler drug, this time fenoterol. The drug's producer, Boehringer Ingelheim, launched a vicious campaign of misinformation against Pearce, and against the notion that their drugs had caused asthma deaths. However, over a three year period, the market share for *fenoterol* dropped from 30% to less than 3%, and the asthma deaths plummeted in line with this drop. See page 178 for an explanation of how this inhaler approach to asthma can eventually cause death—in all inhaler brands.

A similar area is the treatment of cough. Over-the-counter remedies are a lucrative market. But a Cochrane systematic review of the randomized trials shows that none of them are effective.[30]

Astra-Syntex pushes an ineffective and dangerous arthritis drug purely for profit

In the 1970's, a Swiss drug company Astra-Syntex, relied on the success of one main product to ensure the company's survival.[31] This was the drug *naproxen* (Naprosyn), used for arthritis. It belongs to a class of drug known as a nonsteroidal anti-inflammatory drug (NSAID).

There is scientific doubt about whether NSAID's do have any anti-inflammatory effect,[31] but it is certain that the drug does have many serious (and some fatal) adverse effects, such as causing death through a bleeding stomach ulcer, or a heart attack; and the drug should be taken with extreme caution. However, Astra-Syntex relied on the sales of this drug to support the company. The standard dose was 500 mg daily, but the company's salespeople were instructed to persuade doctors to use 1000 mg daily, using dose-response charts created by the drug company, with the maximum effect claimed at a dose of 1500 mg. But these charts were found to be incorrect and misleading.[32] Increasing the dose from 250 mg to 1500 mg of naproxen, would net the drug company six times more revenue, but the trial data that the charts were based on, actually showed that increasing the dose this much made no difference to the pain levels felt by the patient. Whereas, the adverse effects of the drug did increase in a linear fashion dependent on dose. Because the potential adverse effects were serious, the drug company's recommendation should have been to use the smallest dose (250 mg). But purely to increase profits, a higher dose was pushed for, despite the risks to the patient—and also the company's own data that showed that there was no increase in benefit.

A 1986 study[33] of patients with ankle swelling showed that *naproxen* had no effect on the swelling, but that simply encouraging the patients to move around normally, decreased the swelling and they recovered faster. And a 1990 study showed that NSAID'S had no effect on swollen finger joints.[32]

Drug companies make millions by lying about the effectiveness of NSAID's and ignoring the dangers

Pfizer, which eventually became the largest drug company in the world, relied on particularly aggressive and ruthless marketing.[34] That company's NSAID was piroxicam (Feldene), and they lied that it was more effective than aspirin and had a lower rate of gastrointestinal adverse effects than other NSAIDs.[35] However, piroxicam had more fatal reactions and more fatal gastrointestinal adverse effects than other drugs. The BMJ published a paper that demonstrated the high incidence of severe ulcer disease with piroxicam,[36] which Pfizer had attempted to dissuade them from publishing.

Another big drug company, Eli Lilly, knew about the dreadful adverse effects of their NSAID, benoxaprofen (Opren or Oraflex), yet they still aggressively marketed it.[35] The company knew about liver failure and deaths caused by their drug but failed to inform the regulators. A later court case described this as "standard practice in the industry."[37,38] The company published a paper in the BMJ, claiming that no cases of jaundice or deaths had been reported on the drug, which was untrue.[35] Benoxaprofen also caused other unpleasant adverse effects in

10% of patients, including sensitivity to light and loosening of the nails. The elderly were a significant portion of the market and when researchers found that the drug accumulated in the elderly, making it even more toxic, Lilly tried to prevent the study from being published. After fatalities in the elderly, caused by this drug, it was eventually withdrawn.

Roche covered up serious harms in its flu drug and misled governments about its effectiveness

In 2009, Roche convinced US and European governments to stockpile its Tamiflu drug in preparation for that year's expected influenza epidemic, at the cost of billions of dollars and Euros. Roche claimed that the drug reduced hospital admissions by 61%.[39] But this was based on the company's internal trials, which they declined to publish, and attempts by independent Cochrane researchers to access this data were rigorously resisted by Roche. The FDA warned Roche to stop making unsubstantiated claims about the drug,[40, 41] but still approved Tamiflu.

A similar drug, zanamivir, from GlaxoSmithKline, was initially refused approval by the FDA.[42] The drug was found to be no better than placebo[42] (in other words, it did not work), but Glaxo put pressure on the FDA[43] and the drug was approved. Following this pressure, it was later the same year that the FDA also approved Tamiflu, despite there being no convincing evidence that Tamiflu prevented influenza complications. And Tamiflu also had important adverse effects, which were concealed. Roche's own data revealed that cases of hallucinations and weird accidents were fairly commonly reported to them.[44] This was consistent with studies in Japan, where rats exhibited similar symptoms. However, a journal article written by Roche authors claimed that rats and mice were given a high dose of Tamiflu and showed no ill effect, but according to data from Roche's Japanese subsidiary, the same dose of Tamiflu was given to rats, and the drug killed more than half the animals.[44]

5. The conduct of drug companies

Johnson & Johnson concealed the serious risks of its drug

In 2009, Johnson & Johnson paid $75 million to settle corruption charges. It was alleged that they bribed doctors in Greece, Poland and Romania to use the company's products, and bribed hospital administrators in Poland to award them contracts.[45]

In 2012, Johnson & Johnson was fined more than $1.1 billion. They were found to have downplayed and hidden risks associated with its drug Risperdal (an anti-psychotic). It was found that a subsidiary company, Janssen, had lied about potentially life-threatening adverse effects of the drug, which included death, strokes, seizures, weight gain and diabetes.[46] And more than a quarter of the drug's users were children and adolescents.[47] The judge also found nearly 240,000 instances of Medicaid fraud. Further allegations made by the US government in April 2012 were that Johnson & Johnson paid kickbacks to induce the nation's largest nursing home pharmacy, Omnicare, to purchase and recommend Risperdal.[48] This was despite the fact that the FDA had previously rejected the company's attempt to get approval to market Risperdal for treatment of behavioural disturbances in dementia because of safety concerns; and the FDA had warned the drug company that marketing Risperdal as safe and effective in the elderly would be false and misleading.

Pfizer guilty of bribery and fraud on an unprecedented scale

In 2004, Pfizer was fined $430 million after pleading guilty to paying doctors to prescribe its epilepsy drug Neurontin.[76]

In 2009, Pfizer paid $2.3 billion, which was then the largest healthcare fraud settlement in history.[49] In relation to four Pfizer drugs (Bextra, an anti-arthritis drug; Geodon, an antipsychotic; Zyvox, an antibiotic; and Lyrica, an epilepsy drug), the company's subsidiary pleaded guilty to misbranding the drugs "with the intent to defraud or mislead." Pfizer also paid bribes and offered lavish hospitality to healthcare providers to encourage them to prescribe these four drugs. In Pfizer's own fact book, it admitted that the generic antibiotic drug, vancomycin, was a better drug then their own antibiotic, Zyvox. However, they priced their own drug at eight times higher than the generic drug and lied to doctors and hospitals that their drug was better. Due to serious safety concerns, the FDA told Pfizer to stop making its unsubstantiated claims, but Pfizer continued to lie to doctors that their drug would save more lives.[50]

In 2012, a US federal investigation into medical bribery overseas, accused Pfizer of bribing doctors, hospital administrators and drug regulators in Europe and Asia, and of trying to hide the bribery by listing the payments in their accounts as training, freight and entertainment expenses.[51] Court papers also stated that the company wired monthly payments to a doctor in Croatia who helped the government decide which drugs to register. Pfizer paid $60 million to settle the case.

Sanofi-Aventis conducted fraudulent trial of its anti-biotic which caused liver damage

In 2007, the FDA criticized Sanofi-Aventis for failing to act on known instances of fraud during a pivotal trial of its drug Ketex (an antibiotic).[52] One of the doctors involved was convicted of fraud. He claimed to have enrolled over 400 patients to the trial, being paid $400 per patient by the drug company. He faked consent forms for non-existent participants. The FDA also referred three other sites in the trial for criminal investigations.[53] Despite the FDA knowing about the suspect data in the trial, it still approved the drug. When 23 cases of severe liver injury and four deaths had been caused by the drug, the FDA prohibited its scientists to discuss the drug with the media. 16 months after the first case of liver damage became public, the FDA simply relabelled the drug to indicate it was toxic to the liver.[54]

Pushing drugs for non-approved uses

Novartis illegally markets drugs, and bribes doctors to prescribe them

In 2010, Novartis was accused of illegally marketing their drug Trileptal for uses it was not approved for; and also of paying kickbacks to healthcare professionals to induce them to prescribe this, and also five other of the company's drugs. Novartis paid $420 million to settle the case.[55]

Eli Lilly guilty of illegal marketing tactics to sell an unapproved drug with serious adverse effects

In 2005, Eli Lilly paid $36 million to settle criminal charges related to their drug Evista (a drug intended for osteoporosis). The charges were that they concealed data that the drug showed an increased risk of ovarian cancer; then they illegally marketed the drug for prevention of breast cancer and heart disease.[56]

In 2009, Eli Lilly were fined more than $1.4 billion for illegal marketing, after pleading guilty to criminal charges. This concerned their drug Zyprexa (an anti-psychotic); it was already a top-selling drug, but they illegally marketed it for a wide range of conditions that it was not approved for, including Alzheimer's, depression and dementia, focusing on children and the elderly, despite the fact that the drug's adverse effects are substantial: inducing heart failure, pneumonia, considerable weight gain and diabetes. They gave lectures and conferences for physicians, and planted their own sales people in the audience to ask scripted questions, designed to encourage the use of the drug for these unapproved conditions. Zyprexa made worldwide sales of $40 billion between 1996 and 2009,[57] so that the $1.4 billion fine was no disincentive. Using illegal methods to boost sales, regardless of the harm and fatalities caused, is clearly commercially lucrative. This may explain why profit appears to trump morality in pharmaceutical corporations.

Sanofi-Aventis uses fraud to boost profits even more

In 2009, Sanofi-Aventis was charged with fraud. Between 1995 and 2000 the drug company deliberately misquoted prices, to underpay rebates to Medicaid and overcharge public health agencies for their drugs. To settle the fraud charge, the drug company paid $95 million.[58]

GlaxoSmithKline guilty of selling unapproved drugs, bribing doctors, and covering up serious adverse effects of their diabetes drug

In 2003, GlaxoSmithKline was fined $88 million for overcharging Medicaid for their drugs Paxil and Flonase.[59]

In 2003, the Inland Revenue Service made a claim against GlaxoSmithKline for $7.8 billion in backdated taxes. And in 2006, the company paid another $3.1 billion to settle a tax dispute relating to their policy of moving money between different companies.[59]

In 2004, GlaxoSmithKline was accused of corruption in Italy, in a €228 million scheme involving 73 company employees who had bribed 4,000 Italian doctors to induce them to prescribe the company's products.[60]

In 2009, GlaxoSmithKline was fined $750 million for fraud.[61] Their manufacturing plant in Puerto Rico was closed down due to it producing adulterated drugs. The company's quality assurance manager raised concerns with the company and she was fired.[62] And Glaxo lied to federal investigators about the problems, despite the company receiving complaints direct from pharmacies.

In 2011, GlaxoSmithKline paid $3 billion to settle a fraud case, which is the largest fraud settlement in US history.[63] Glaxo pleaded guilty to illegally marketing a number of drugs for uses they were not approved for, including Wellbutrin and Paxil (antidepressants), Advair (an asthma drug), Avandia (a diabetes drug), and Lamictal (an epilepsy drug). The company also paid kickbacks to doctors and failed to include certain safety data in reports to the FDA. Also, the FDA-approved label for Avandia warned of the cardiovascular risks associated with the drug, but GlaxoSmithKline's promotional programmes suggested the drug had cardiovascular benefits. In Europe, the drug was withdrawn because it increased cardiovascular deaths.

AstraZeneca markets unapproved drug for children and the elderly, and bribes doctors

In 2003, AstraZeneca were fined $520 million for fraud. They bribed doctors to buy their drug Zoladex (for prostate cancer) then illegally encouraged them to request Medicare reimbursements for the drug.[64]

In 2010, AstraZeneca paid $520 million to settle further fraud charges. They were accused of marketing Seroquel (an anti-psychotic drug) for uses it was not approved for. They targeted children, the elderly, veterans and inmates, marketing the drug for aggression, Alzheimer's, anger management, anxiety, dementia, depression, etc., though the drug was not approved for these uses.[65] The company paid kickbacks and other incentives (such as lavish holidays) to doctors to encourage them to prescribe the drug for these purposes.

Massive though these fines are, they are no disincentive to drug companies, as the profits from such activities far outweigh the fines. This particular drug, Seroquel, made $4.9 billion in 2009 alone,[66] which is more than nine times the fine. In other words, a single year's profits are not notably dented by such fines, and the profits role in, year after year. The temptation to chase profits, despite the detriment to patients' healthcare, is obvious.

Defrauding taxpayers and bribing doctors

Merck guilty of defrauding taxpayers, and bribing doctors

In 2007, Merck were ordered to pay $670 million in relation to Medicade fraud. They also paid kickbacks to doctors and hospitals to induce them to prescribe their drugs.[67] From 1997 to 2001, Merck's sales force used fifteen different programmes to induce doctors to prescribe its drugs, which consisted of making excess payments to doctors disguised as fees for "training", "consultation" or "market research."

Abbott covered up adverse effects of their drug, then illegally marketed it to the very patients most at risk of those effects

In 2012, Abbott were fined $1.5 billion for Medicaid fraud, concerning their drug Depakote (an epilepsy drug).[68] The company halted a trial of the drug in elderly, demented patients because of increasing adverse effects; then Abbott laboratories made false and misleading statements about the safety, effectiveness, and cost effectiveness of the drug for use in elderly, demented patients (which it was not approved for), while paying kickbacks to doctors to induce them to prescribe or promote the drug.

Abbott and Takeda defraud taxpayers, and use improper sales practices

In 2001, TAP Pharmaceuticals (Abbott and Takeda) were fined $875 million for fraud. They gave drugs to doctors for free or at a reduced price, then encouraged them to bill the government for the full price.[69,70] In 2003, Abbott paid $622 million to settle an investigation into their sales practices.[69]

To sell their products, drug companies routinely use bribery and covering up of serious adverse effects

In 2007 Bristol-Myers Squibb paid $515 million to settle allegations of illegal marketing and fraudulent pricing practices, involving payments to doctors do induce them to use the company's drugs, and to also use them for conditions they were not approved for.[71]

In 2007, Purdur Pharma was fined $635 million. To boost sales of their drug OxyContin (similar to morphine) they lied to doctors that their drug was less addictive, less subject to abuse, and had less withdrawal symptoms than other opiates. The drug became popular among drug abusers, killing a huge number of users; and many legitimate users died due to accidental overdosing.[72]

5. The conduct of drug companies

In 2006, it was revealed in a US lawsuit that Medtronic had spent at least $50 million over four years, on bribes to back surgeons. One surgeon alone was paid nearly $700,000 in nine months.[73] They paid between $1,000 and $2,000 for each patient who was implanted with one of the company's devices.[74]

In 2007, five manufacturers of hip and knee replacements admitted bribing surgeons to use their products. The bribes ranged from tens to hundreds of thousands of dollars per year. The companies involved were Zimmer, DePuy Orthopaedics, Biomet, Smith & Nephew, and Stryker Orthopaedics.[75]

In 2006, Serono Laboratories were fined $704 million after pleading guilty to using an elaborate scheme of bribery to encourage the use of its AIDS drug, Serostim.[76]

It should be stated that many of the crimes committed by drug companies are only possible because of the active cooperation of doctors, who are rarely punished for their role.

In 2004, a British government Health Committee examined the drug industry in detail and found that its influence was enormous and out of control.[77] They found that drug companies buy influence over doctors, charities, journalists and politicians, and that regulation of drug companies is sometimes weak or ambiguous.[78]

In 1970, the US produced legislation aimed at countering organised crime, its centrepiece being the Racketeer Influenced and Corrupt Organizations Act (RICO).[79] Under the definitions of this act, the routine activities of the pharmaceutical industry meet all the main criteria for organized crime. Peter Rost, former vice president of marketing for Pfizer, also compares drug industries to the mob. He says that both make obscene amounts of money; in both, the side effects of their activities are killings and death; and both bribe politicians and others.[80]

6. Can the reported outcome of a drug trial be taken at face value?

Marcia Angell, editor of the New England Journal of Medicine for 20 years, said "It is simply no longer possible to believe much of the clinical research that is published, or to rely on the judgement of trusted physicians or authoritative medical guidelines."[1] This chapter provides insights into some of the dishonest methods used by drug companies to produce fraudulent drug-trial outcomes to sell their products.

Does the "placebo effect" really exist?

A drug trial is supposed to find out if a drug is effective at improving a particular condition, and does not harm the patient (the drug's adverse effects). But it is not easy to determine if a drug has any positive effect. In many trials, half the patients take the drug, while the other half take a pill that has no effect, but none of the participants (including the doctors) are supposed to know which pill each patient is taking (the trial is then "blind", or "double blind" if neither the patient nor doctors know which pill each patient took). It is usually found that in the patients who take the inert pill, the condition being treated can improve markedly. This has become known as the placebo effect. The theory is that just because the patient *thinks* they are being treated, this causes their mind to somehow heal their condition.

For example, in trials of anti-depressants where patients take either the drug or a placebo pill for six weeks, it is often found that about 60% of the people taking the drug, show some improvement in their condition. But around 50% of the people taking the placebo pill also show an improvement in their condition.[2]

Due to results like this, it is now generally believed that the placebo effect can be substantial in many people. At least, this is the interpretation that drug companies would like us to believe.

Why Use Natural Healing?

The implication of the above trials is that among the 60% of the people who took the drug and improved, in 50% of these people the improvement was due to the placebo effect. This is because the placebo effect is also imaged to exist even when people take an active drug. Therefore, the drug is thought to have a genuine positive effect in only 10% of the people who take it.

But mainstream healthcare believes that the placebo effect is powerful, and if this can produce an improvement in 50% of people (some medics even claim it works in 70% of people), then the thinking is that it is worthwhile prescribing a drug that only has an effect in 10% of people, because when the placebo effect is added to this, then 60% (or even 80%) of people who take the drug will improve.

However, it has been shown that the placebo effect is either minimal, or does not exist at all.[3,4] In trials like the above, where the condition improved after six weeks in 50% of the participants who took no active drug, this was due to the condition simply improving by itself with no treatment. This is known as spontaneous remission, or the natural course of the disease. But this is bad news for drug companies, because if their trials show that their drug will only have an effect in 10% of people who take it, but in at least 50% of people, the condition would improve by itself when they take no drug at all, then it is difficult to justify subjecting 100% of people to the drug's adverse effects, which can often be severe. Therefore drug companies choose to portray the placebo effect as real and powerful, which then justifies doctors prescribing their drugs, to hopefully trigger the imaginary placebo effect.

In other words, according to the science, most patients would be better off taking no drugs at all, and not even attending a doctor (p.108). But drug companies use various tactics to conceal this knowledge from doctors and the public. This invented "placebo effect" is just one such tactic.

Is there a statistical slight of hand?

The results of drug trials are usually reported with a "P" value. When a P value is 0.04 or less, the results are then said to be "statistically significant". What does this mean? Most people, including most doctors, have no idea what this really means. Therefore, they have no choice but to accept that the trial "proved" the drug works.

A P value means the percent probability that the improvement noticed was real and did not merely happen by chance. Even though the noticed improvement only occurred in a small number of people who took part in the trial, a P value provides a way of deciding if the effect was real, or whether it was just a chance occurrence. If the improvement happened by chance and the trial were repeated many times, the same improvements would not occur. But trials cannot be repeated many times, due to the expense and opportunity, so the P value provides a way of performing this test statistically.

When $P = 0.04$, this means there is a 4% probability that the result happened by chance; or a 96% probability that the results were real. This is considered enough to "prove" that the results were real. Hence the results are said to be "statistically significant", meaning that from a statistical point of view, the claimed results were not due to chance. Therefore it is assumed that the drug does have the effect that was noticed (even though it only occurred in 10%, or even less, of people in the trial).

How small a change is needed in the trial results to affect the P value?

Peter Gøtzsche gives the following example. Suppose a trial were conducted using 400 patients, who were randomly placed into two groups, one taking the active drug and the other taking a placebo pill. If 60% of the active group (121 patients) improved, and 50% of the placebo group (100 patients) improved, this would produce a P value of 0.04. In other words, there is a 96% probability that the results were real, rather than occurred by chance. The results would be considered "statistically significant" and this would be taken as "proof" that the drug worked. But if two fewer patients had improved on the active drug (119, instead of 121 patients), then the P value would become 0.07, and it could not be claimed that the results were "statistically significant", and therefore the results would not have "proved" that the drug worked.[5]

For drug companies, when a trial does not prove that a drug works, it is far too tempting to re-analyze the data, and now find that two more patients had improved on the active drug, or two less patients had improved on the placebo pill, or to exclude some patients from the analysis. These new results would then be "statistically significant" and be taken as "proof" that the drug works.

It has been demonstrated through criminal trials of drug companies that this type of data-tampering is routinely performed (pp.63-67).[6] In this situation, drug trial results can be considered no more than a marketing smoke screen.

Other errors inherent in many trials

But even when such drug-trial tampering is not consciously done, the same distortion of the data can easily occur unintentionally. Trials are usually intended to be either blind (where the patient did not know whether they took an active drug or a placebo pill) or double blind (where neither the doctor nor patient knew this). If the blinding is secure, when the patient or the doctor evaluate the improvement in the patient, the results can be considered more reliable. But the blinding is far too easily broken. For example, many drugs have notable adverse effects, which would reveal to both the patient and doctor that the patient had taken the active drug and not the placebo. This would then cause a bias when the patient's improvement was assessed.

It has been shown that in trials where a non-blinded observer evaluated the results, the effect of the improvement in the patient who was known to have taken the active drug, was exaggerated by 36%.[7] This means that in a trial that was supposed to be double blind, the improvement in the patients who took the active drug could be substantially exaggerated. When many drugs are found to only produce an improvement in about 10% of the people who take it, this degree of bias (up to 36% exaggeration of improvement), can make the results of the trial meaningless. And as shown in the above example of a trial using 400 participants (p.81), only a small change in the outcomes of two

6. Can the reported outcome of a drug trial be taken at face value?

of those patients was needed to turn the trial results from negative to positive. Hence, bias due to the blinding being broken can turn a negative result into a positive one, and thus "prove" that a drug worked, when it was actually not proven to work.

An attempt to solve this problem was made with the creation of an active placebo. This is a pill that produces one of the adverse effects that the test drug would produce, but does not include the active drug itself. For example, a common adverse effect of an anti-depressant is that it produces dryness of the mouth; and trials have been performed where the placebo pill contained atropine, which causes dryness of the mouth. This would have convinced many of the participants that they were taking the active drug, therefore this removed the usual bias that is introduced when assessing the improvement, because the participants who took the active drug could not be distinguished from those who took the placebo pill.

In such trials, there was a considerably smaller difference in the outcomes between the two groups when compared to trials that did not use an active placebo.[8] In other words, even though the usual trials may only show an improvement in about 10% of the patients who took the active drug, when bias was removed, the drug was shown to only work in far fewer than 10% of the people who took it.

In response to this, the drug companies declined to produce active placebo pills for trials. From the commercial point of view, their reasoning is clear: why should they assist researchers to demonstrate that their drugs don't work? But beyond this, drug companies also refuse to produce inactive placebo pills for use in trials of their drugs.[9] A placebo pill should look and have the same texture and weight as the active drug. Or on occasions, when they agree to produce such a pill, they quote such an astronomical price for it that the trial cannot proceed.[9] This ensures that "placebo controlled" trials remain under the control of the drug company who produce the drug; they decide how a trial is designed, whether the trial results are made public, and have complete control over how the data is analysed; and the data then becomes the property of the drug company, who usually refuse to release it to the public (for "commercial" reasons), unless compelled to through litigation.

Why are drugs designed for one purpose but often marketed for many other purposes?

All the flaws described in drug trials (including bias reporting by non-blinded assessors, and data manipulation), explain why it is so easy for a drug company to take one of its drugs, designed to improve a particular condition, and trial that drug for several other conditions, and manage to produce a trial outcome that "proves" that the drug works for these other conditions, even when in reality, the drug has no effect whatsoever on those conditions. The downside of this practice, apart from the expense to the patient and health service, is that patients are subjected to all the adverse effects of the drug, with no possible positive effect of taking the drug. Pages 72-75 give many proven examples of this practice.

Other dishonest methods used to manipulate drug trials to produce misleading results

Rather than using an honest, scientific approach, it has become standard practice for drug companies to manipulate many aspects of drug trials, simply to produce false and misleading outcomes whose only purpose is to sell their products, with complete disregard for the health of their customers. Apart from the dishonesty covered so far, the following are further devices used to produce misleading trial outcomes that favour the drug company.

The trial data is kept secret

When a trial is sponsored by a drug company, it is usual for the drug company to require ownership of the data, and also to demand that they must approve the manuscript before it may be published.[10] This means that the data would be protected from being made public (so that any manipulation of the data may not be scrutinized), and if the drug company is not happy with the outcome of the trial, they would be able to block its publication.

An internal AstraZeneca email[11] (which was released due to court proceedings), commented on these routine practices amongst its competitor drug companies: "...Lilly offer significant financial support [for trials] but want control of the data in return. They are able to spin the same data in many different ways through an effective publication team. Negative data usually remains well hidden.... most proposals [for research projects] are modified by Bristol-Myers Squibb. Strategic focus is unlicensed indications [i.e. to obtain data to be used in marketing to doctors, to persuade them to use their drugs for unapproved conditions, and hence greatly boost profit] ... no [trial] data is allowed to be published without going through Janssen for approval, and communication is controlled by Janssen... investigators who publish favourable results... are well rewarded for their involvement."

Halting trials prematurely

Another method used by drug companies is to stop a trial prematurely. When the data gathered so far reflects well on the drug being tested, the trial is halted at that point because if the trial were permitted to run its full length, the true results may reflect poorly on the drug being tested. It was found that trials that were stopped early in this way, tended to exaggerate the treatment effect of the trial drug by 39%, compared to trials that were not stopped early.[12] It is common for drug companies to specify in the trial protocol that they have the right to stop a trial at any time and for any reason.

Currently, in both Europe and the US, most trials of drugs are sponsored by the companies that manufacture and market the drugs;[13] and the research is mostly (74%) carried out by private companies with close connections to the drug companies (and also with advertising and marketing firms), rather than by academic institutions.[14]

Drug companies also change trial protocols to conceal harms, and manufacture a fake positive outcome

Another common way for drug companies to cheat is this. Before a drug trial takes place, a protocol is produced. This defines the outcomes that the trial is designed to test for. For example, the trial may be intended to test the company's new drug against an already existing drug, and to determine which is more effective at making an improvement in a certain condition; or which has less adverse effects of a certain type (for example, which drug accidentally causes more heart attacks, drug A or drug B?). But when all the data has been gathered and is analysed, this provides drug companies with another easy way to cheat. If the results prove that their new drug causes more heart attacks than their competitor's existing drug, then the company would simply change the trial protocol, and pretend the trial was testing for a different factor. This would then conceal the negative data, which condemned their own, new drug (for many examples of this, see page 92). And instead, they analyse the data again in many different ways, until they find an outcome that is positive for their drug, and this is the trial that is published. In this case, the trial would not now even mention heart attacks, and if that issue comes up in future law suits, the company is able to claim that their trial did not test for heart attacks, and simply lie that they have not seen any data that suggests their drug causes heart attacks. The new protocol would claim to be testing for some other factor, which the data came out positive for when they analysed the results after the trial. For example, there may be a positive result for their new drug producing an improvement in a particular symptom. In this case, the drug would be marketed as improving this symptom, and no mention would be made of the fact that the drug accidentally causes heart attacks. The hope would be that by the time this is discovered (several years later), the company would have already made many billions from the drug.

In 2004, 102 protocols were studied from published trials. About 75% of the trials were sponsored by drug companies, and the remainder were independent. It was found that in 63% of the trials, the primary outcome had been changed from that in the original protocol, and in 33% of the trials a new primary outcome appeared in the published trial, which did not even exist in the original protocol. In 71% of the trials, there was at least one outcome defined in the protocol which was not reported when the trial was published; but in all these trials, missing from the published version of the trial, there was an average of four outcomes related to effectiveness, and three outcomes that measured major adverse effects. All these were defined in the original protocols; hence the trials looked for these outcomes; but after the results were analysed, it may be surmised that a decision was taken to not publish these outcomes, since they would have a negative (or even fatal) impact on the drug's marketing.[15]

Conclusion

The inference of this (and the previous) chapter is that when drug companies produce a new drug, they often realize that they do not have a viable product. Their own trials have shown that the drug does not work, and only has many adverse effects. But drug companies are massive corporations, whose sole aim is to continue to make massive profits. Therefore, they need to falsify the trial results and cover up the worst of the adverse effects, in order to be able to sell their product.

Because their only real goal is to make money, they are not concerned about healthcare in general, or about how many people's lives are ruined by their drugs. To them, that is simply the acceptable consequence of obtaining big profits; and from a commercial point of view, the fines for their criminal actions are tiny when compared to the profits (see Chapter 5), so law suits are just a minor irritant

In order to survive, it appears that drug companies have realized that they cannot allow their drugs to be properly tested by independent scientific methods, because this would demonstrate that the drugs have no beneficial effect and many harmful adverse effects; and they would then have no product to sell in the lucrative markets that they themselves have created and have become accustomed to profiting from.

Even vitamins can be harmful

In 2008, a review of the placebo-controlled trials of antioxidants, including beta-carotene, vitamin A and E, showed that taking these supplements increased overall mortality. In other words, whether you are healthy or ill, taking these supplements only shortened your life expectancy.[16]

7. How are useless and harmful drugs pushed?

Once a new drug is produced, it may frequently be found to have no positive effect, but a range of harmful effects, some potentially fatal. This information, the drug company usually carefully conceals. Such products may make up the bulk of a drug company's output. Once they know a drug does not work and is only harmful, and they have covered up this information, they are then only in the business of generating profits—using any means. This has nothing to do with medicine, and is knowingly detrimental to global healthcare. How do they market and push these mercenary drugs?

First, produce a fraudulent trial

The first stage is to produce a fraudulent "trial", with manipulated data and procedures that all produce false claims for the drug, and hide its harmful effects (page 92 onwards gives many examples of such data manipulation by drug companies). This is then used as a key marketing tool. Internal Pfizer documents revealed that they consider "trials" to be merely tools for marketing; for misleading the drug regulators; and for persuading doctors to prescribe their drugs for purposes they are not approved for (simply to explode the profits even further).[1]

But the most important part of the marketing is aimed directly at doctors, which even includes bribes to doctors to help push these mercenary drugs (which make up the bulk of the industry, and the vast majority of a doctor's prescriptions).

Then, bribe the doctors

Doctors are routinely bribed by drug companies to prescribe its drugs. For example, in the small country of Denmark alone, in 2010, over 4,000 doctors were registered as receiving such money directly from drug companies. The bribes were hidden by calling them fees for "advice", helping as an "investigator", and so on.[2] Some naïve doctors may think that the fee is genuinely being paid to them for information they supply and that since drug companies are so rich, they pay a high fee for doing almost nothing. But the "fee" is a thinly disguised bribe. (See pages 75-79 for many more examples of such bribery.)

Another common form of bribery is to recruit doctors in a so-called "seeding trial". The drug company pretends that it is conducting a trial. A "new" drug is produced (see below). Doctors are then paid to enrol their patients into the pretend trial (a German survey found that two-thirds of such trials didn't even have a study plan or an aim for the so-called study[3]). But the real intention is simply to encourage the prescription of this "new" drug, since "modern" drugs are better than the old, much cheaper ones currently in use (which is how the sales spin usually goes). The enrolment fee, of course, is simply a bribe. In such a "seeding trial" by AstraZeneca, doctors were paid $800 for each patient they enrolled in the pretend trial. This resulted in a significant increase in the use of the company's drugs in the doctors' practices.[4]

The intentions of the drug company (in this and in making bribes in other forms) was made clear by internal documents: "When a gift or gesture of any size is bestowed [on doctors], it imposes on the recipient a sense of indebtedness. The obligation to directly reciprocate tends to influence behaviour. Food, flattery and friendship are powerful tools of persuasion, particularly when combined."[5]

Another form of bribery is so-called consultancy fees. In countries with a large drug market, drug companies hire many thousands of doctors as "consultants", often paying substantial fees. The doctors chosen are key "opinion leaders", as they exert considerable influence on which drugs other specialists and general practitioners use. The large reward is simply a bribe to the doctor to promote the drug company's products. In a criminal fraud case against TAP Pharmaceuticals, it was found that their "consultants" never prepared reports or billed TAP for their time; and the sales employees who nominated the "consultants" typically had no discussions with the doctors regarding the consulting services to be provided.[6]

7. How are useless and harmful drugs pushed?

A substantial part of drug company activity consists of producing these "new" drugs that are really not new at all, and are merely slight variations of existing, cheap drugs; and pricing their "new" drug at around ten times more than the existing drug (such drugs cost next to nothing to produce, but they use the standard lie that "it is very expensive to develop these drugs"[7]). To market their new drug, they use all the above tricks to produce fake trial results that claim that their new drug is much more effective, and has less serious adverse effects, than the existing, cheap drug. This produces the false impression that these "new", "modern" drugs are better than the old ones. But in most cases, if the trial had been conducted honestly it often reveals that their "new" drug performs in the same way as the existing, much cheaper drug; or sometimes it does not perform as well.[8] The whole activity is about fraudulently generating as much profit as possible, with no concern for healthcare, or for national healthcare budgets.[9]

After manufacturing fake trial results, misleading articles are then produced to assist in the marketing. The articles are "ghost written" by employees of the drug company,[10] and they praise these "new" drugs, giving false accounts of their benefits and understating their harms. A prominent academic is then handsomely paid to put his name to the article,[11] which is then published in a leading medical journal, and influences doctors to prescribe the drugs.[12]

It has been shown that general practitioners depend on the drug industry as their main source of information about drugs,[13, 14] and that doctors are not able to separate correct from misleading information.[13, 15] Hence, whether or not a patient is prescribed a drug, and which drug they get, is determined entirely by this type of marketing by drug companies. This is even more alarming when the supposed benefit of the drug was made up by the drug company, and its adverse effects were concealed.

Concerning blood-pressure issues, even though the theory is misguided (Chapter 3), when drugs are prescribed, this is often based on fraudulent information from drug companies (see below). In 2002, a blood-pressure related trial was published using 33,357 patients, the ALLHAT trial.[16] It found that the most commonly prescribed drugs were by far the most expensive ones, which had been promoted using false information. And it was estimated that these expensive, "modern" drugs had caused heart failure in 40,000 US patients.

Negative data about drugs is concealed to make the drugs seem effective

Hans Melander is the chief statistician at the Swedish drug agency. In 2003 he compared 42 published trial reports of anti-depressants (SSRI's) with the trial data that the drug companies had submitted to the drug regulation authorities.[17] He found the published reports were seriously flawed, with the drug companies leaving out data that reflected negatively on their drug, so that the published reports portrayed the drugs as being much more effective than they really were.

In 2008, a similar study in the US had the same finding.[18] Because of the data that drug companies had fraudulently withheld from their published trial reports, this made the drugs appear 32% more effective than they really were; and when compared to the trials that the drug companies had withheld from publication completely, the published trials had exaggerated the effectiveness of their drugs by more than 50%. And another 2008 study, of 164 trials submitted to the US FDA by drug companies, found that the trial reports that were eventually made public, did not reflect the trials submitted to the FDA.[19]

Drug regulatory agencies (rather than protecting the public) often appear to collude with drug companies to cover up such fraud. For example, when data that a drug company submitted to them revealed that a drug intended to prevent suicides had actually caused a suicide during the drug's trial, the FDA chose to regard this data as the drug company's trade secret, and refused to publish it.[20]

When drug companies sponsor trials that reflect badly on their drugs, the companies claim that even the very existence of such trials is a trade secret.[21] On average only about 50% of all studies ever get published.[22] And as shown above, many of the published trials do not reflect the actual trial data anyway.

Sanofi-Aventis conceals harms in its drug

In 2007, for the purposes of a study, Peter Gøtzsche requested access to the clinical study reports for rimonabant (an anti-obesity drug).[23] These had been submitted to the European Medicines Agency (EMA) by the drug company, Sanofi-Aventis, and had not been made public. A three year legal battle ensued, with the EMA arguing that the documents could not be revealed because it would undermine the commercial interests of the drug company. In the meantime, the drug was withdrawn from the European market when independent studies found that the adverse effects (including severe depression and increased risk of suicide) were more serious and common than shown in the clinical trials that the drug company *had* published.[24]

Roche conceals suicide-risk of its drug

In 2002, Danish journalists tried to get access to the adverse effects of the drug Roaccutane (an acne drug produced by Roche) that had been reported by Roche to the Danish medical agency. The agency was willing to disclose the data, but this was blocked by Roche who argued that it would create a substantial risk for considerable losses by them; and Roche even threatened to sue the regulator if they disclosed the true nature of the adverse effects of their drug and this harmed their commercial interests (in other words, Roche was convinced it had a right to the huge profits that could only be made by concealing from people the true suicidal risks of its drug).[25] In 2010, Liam Grant (the father of a boy who committed suicide while on this same drug, Roaccutane) applied to the EMA to try to find out which adverse effects Roche had informed them about before marketing approval was granted; and the EMA finally granted access to the data.[26]

Wyeth conceals fatal harms of its slimming pill

In the USA, slimming pills were big business. In 1973, the drug Pondimin was marketed by Wyeth. After many deaths caused by this drug, and continued pressure on Wyeth, the company produced a new pill that combined Pondimin with an older drug (phentermine), calling the new pill Fen-Phen. It became extremely popular. In 1996 alone, prescriptions exceeded 18 million. But by the summer of 1997, 24 women had developed heart valve disease while on Fen-Phen.[27] The FDA then pressed Wyeth to withdraw the drug from the market.[28] But Wyeth rigorously defended their drug with bogus counter-claims that the drug was safe. American Home Products, which marketed Pondimin, had accumulated internal records of 160 cases of women who had developed high blood pressure in the lung arteries (pulmonary hypertension), but they continued to market the drug. In response to legal proceedings related to the drug, the company destroyed thousands of internal documents and emails, and claimed that they had never even promoted the drug. When the plaintiffs' lawyers gained access to Wyeth's archives, they uncovered reports of 101 cases of high blood pressure in the lung arteries, and more than 50 cases of heart valve disease, which Wyeth had concealed by naming them something else.[28] Pondimin was finally withdrawn in 1997 because it caused high blood pressure in the lung arteries, and also disease of the heart valves. Both these diseases are devastating, and at the time of the law suit it was estimated that 45,000 US women were believed to have developed these diseases while on the drug.[28]

Pfizer illegally promotes its epilepsy drug for other non-approved purposes that it had no effect on

In 2004, Pfizer pleaded guilty to two serious criminal charges of fraud, and was fined $430 million. It had fraudulently promoted its epilepsy drug, Neurontin, for many uses it was not approved for.[29] But such fines provide no disincentive for drug companies to behave criminally. During 2003 alone, sales of Neurontin reached $2,700 million, with about 90% of these sales related to the illegal, non-approved uses.[30]

Some of this activity was committed by Warner-Lambert, which was later bought by Pfizer. Articles were written by the drug company to claim that Neurontin worked for conditions it had not been approved for, and doctors were paid to put their names to these articles.[31] Internal documents (obtained during litigation) revealed the extent to which the company distorted the evidence.[32] Their manipulations involved selective statistical analyses, selective reporting of outcomes (only reporting the ones that showed a positive effect), inappropriate exclusions of some patients in the analyses, multiple publication of desirable results, and spin to make negative results appear positive. The trials were also deliberately biased at the design stage, to ensure that the patients and doctors knew when they were taking an actual drug (rather than a placebo), which then biased the reporting of the drug's effect. And the doctors who participated in trials were not permitted to write up the results. The drug company maintained "editorial" control, and would write up the results, ensuring that the "publication messages" were aligned with the company's global marketing efforts. In relation to the illegal marketing charges, the company's publication strategy was revealed to be to only publish positive results, and to hide the negative results by delaying publication for as long as possible. Kay Dickersin, of the independent Cochrane research centre, summarized the company's activities as: "Outright deception of the biomedical community, highly unethical, harmful to science, wasteful of public resources, and potentially dangerous to the public's health." In all the company-sponsored trials she reviewed, she stated that any positive results could be explained by their selective analysis.[33]

Drug company sales people were then permitted to sit in on doctor-patient consultations (the salesperson, in effect, being presented as a medical student), with the salesperson prompting the doctor to prescribe Neurontin for a wide range of conditions.[31] The doctors who were high-volume prescribers were rewarded by the drug company in various ways.[31, 32] The range of unapproved conditions for Neurontin is listed in a drug index called Drugdex, which lists 48 conditions that the drug may be used for (even though unapproved).[31]

In 2010, in relation to Neurontin, Pfizer was fined a further $142 million, after it was found that the company had engaged in a racketeering conspiracy over a ten-year period, which violated the federal Racketeer Influenced and Corrupt Organizations Act (RICO).[34]

In other words, the company produced fraudulent documents claiming their drug was effective for many conditions, but in reality it had no positive effect on any of the conditions. They then bribed thousands of doctors to prescribe the drug. This meant that millions of patients used their expensive drug, received no benefit for their condition but were exposed to all the adverse effects of the drug, some of which were fatal. Victims of this type of unapproved prescribing have died, suffered heart attacks and strokes, had permanent nerve damage or lost their eyesight.[35] Pfizer is not alone in acting like this. Similar examples are described in this book relating to all the major drug companies. The focus is on profit, using whatever improper methods they can dream up, and there is a total disregard for healthcare. The comparisons with organized crime are apt.

Merck manipulated data to conceal serious harms in their arthritis drug

From 1999, Merck sold their drug Vioxx, an anti-arthritis drug. From their own trials, they knew the drug caused thrombosis,[36] and that it increased the risk of heart attack, but they concealed these facts by data manipulation and careful trial design.[37] Merck conducted two trials[38,39] which both showed the drug increased heart attacks and related conditions. But they delayed the publication of these trials until two years after they had been forced to withdraw the drug from the market (which meant that the truth could no longer affect sales). In one of these trials,[39] three heart attacks in the trial participants were omitted from the trial report, which changed the reported outcome considerably. And in the data that Merck submitted to the FDA, a further death from heart attack was concealed by calling it something else; and many more adverse effects were concealed in the published trial report.[40] In 2007, Merck paid $4.85 billion to settle claims for damages caused by Vioxx,[41] after spending more than $1.2 billion on its own legal fees to fight these claims.[42] And in 2012, Merck pleaded guilty to criminal charges related to its promotion and marketing of Vioxx, and were fined $321.6 million.[43] The crimes involved making false statements about the drug's safety, and marketing the drug for conditions it was not approved for (this included around 30 conditions,[44] suggesting that Merck was marketing the drug as a cure-all, despite knowing about its potentially fatal adverse effects). It has been estimated that Vioxx has killed around 120,000 people.[45]

Pfizer subsidiary manipulated data to conceal serious harms in its drugs

A class of drugs known as non-steroidal anti-inflammatory drugs (NSAID's) is a massive market. To take advantage of this market, a company called Pharmacia (now owned by Pfizer), produced a new NSAID, called Celebrex. A known concern with NSAID's is that they increase the risk of death from stomach ulcers and heart attacks. Pharmacia's own trials of their new drug showed that it was no better than the existing and much cheaper NSAIDS in this respect. But to pretend their drug was much safer than the existing drugs, the company produced a fraudulent trial by "cherry picking" data from two separate trials and presenting it as though it came from a single trial, then "massaging" the data to produce the outcome they wanted (these descriptions of "cherry picked" and "massaged" were made by medical directors from the drug company itself[46]). The two original trials ran for 12 and 15 months, and the fraudulent trail was claimed to have run for 6 months.[47] The fraudulent trial report was published in 2000,[48] and claimed that Celebrex resulted in fewer stomach ulcers than the two existing drugs it was compared with, diclofenac and ibuprofen. But when the data from the two original trials was analysed by independent researchers, this claimed advantage of Celebrex disappeared.[49] And when the FDA examined the complete, original data, it concluded that Celebrex exhibited no advantage in reducing ulcer complications over the two old, much cheaper drugs.[50] But the fraudulent trial did the trick, and by 2004 Celebrex was among the top 10 selling drugs in the US.[51]

In 2005, a trial of Celebrex was ended prematurely for safety concerns, as the drug significantly increased heart and circulatory problems.[52] And in 2006, an analysis conducted by the FDA showed that Celebrex doubled the number of heart attacks in patients who took the drug.[53] It has been estimated that up to 2004, Celebrex had caused 70,000 deaths in the US due to thrombosis, and killed many thousands of patients due to ulcer complications.[54] A 2004 study showed that the bombardment of doctors by drug companies claiming that their new NSAID'S have fewer gastrointestinal adverse effects than the existing NSAIDS, only exacerbated the problems caused by these drugs. Previously the hospital admissions for gastrointestinal bleeding had been decreasing, but as the total sales of all NSAIDS increased (including Celebrex), these hospital admissions started to increase.[55] It is estimated that 3,700 deaths are caused in the UK each year due to peptic ulcer complications in users of NSAID's,[56] which corresponds to around 20,000 annual deaths in the US.

GlaxoSmithKline concealed fatal harms in their drug

In 1999, SmithKline Beecham produced an anti-diabetic drug called Avandia (rosiglitazone). The FDA (who were under pressure from a diabetic patient group) approved the drug, even though they knew it produced blood clots within the heart blood vessels. In a trial conducted by the drug company, the drug also produced more cardiac problems than a competing drug (pioglitazone). The company decided that their "data should not see the light of day to anyone outside of GSK,"[57,58] and they spent the next eleven years trying to cover up this information.[58]

By 2006, Avandia was the top selling diabetes drug worldwide. But in 2007, due to a fraud investigation of Glaxo (in relation to its drug, paroxetine), the company was compelled to publish the results of its clinical trials on a website.[57,59] When independent researchers examined the data for Avandia, the data showed that the drug caused heart attacks and death.[60,61] The drug company had known about this for eight years but had failed to alert the regulatory authorities. It was a US Senate Finance Committee that uncovered the extensive measures that Glaxo had taken to cover up the harms of their drug.[61]

By 2010, the drug was suspended in Europe, but in the US, the FDA still permitted the drug to be used. In 2009, Glaxo attemped to start a six year trial of the drug in the US or Europe, but doctors were unwilling to enrol patients (the trial was unethical), so the trial was begun in India, only to be halted in 2010 by the Indian regulator. Two FDA safety officers had suggested stopping the trial, since it was unethical and the drug caused 500 heart attacks and 300 cases of heart failure every month in the US.[62]

Conclusion

In drug trials carried out by drug companies, it is common (almost universal) for the companies to cheat in various ways, so as to produce a trial report that claims to prove the effectiveness of their drug. When such trials are carried out in good faith, a negative result can kill the drug before it is even marketed. Whereas a fraudulent positive result, can earn the company billions of dollars in the world markets. The incentive to cheat is obvious. This colossal revenue is earned by making just a few dishonest adjustments to the figures when the trial data is analysed by the drug company. And drug companies have demonstrated repeatedly that they are not concerned about the welfare of patients; they are all about making money, and as much as possible, by whatever means they can get away with. And even when they are found out and fined, the fine is usually a small fraction of the profits they make from that same drug. So even using dishonest methods that they know may be eventually discovered and proved in a court of law, is no disincentive. Therefore, any methods whatsoever are open for them to use, which they do.

8. Drug companies create fictitious illnesses to boost profits

Another method used by drug companies purely to boost profits, is to invent an illness, so that their drug can be prescribed for it. And it is usually the case that the drug has no real benefit for the person (as described earlier), but is only detrimental to their health, in the short and long term.

This method has been used extensively in the area of psychiatry. In the US, The Diagnostic and Statistical Manual of Mental Disorders (DSM), now lists 374 mental conditions, all of which may be "medicated" for. For example, women who are beaten by their husbands are declared to have Masochistic Personality Disorder (and require "medicating"). And a man who is unable to establish and maintain a meaningful interpersonal relationship, is declared to have Delusional Dominating Personality Disorder (and requires "medicating"). Normal children could be labelled as having Oppositional Defiant Disorder (and require "medicating"). Normal women could be labelled as having Defeating Personality Disorder (and require "medicating"); or Premenstrual Dysphoric Disorder (and, of course, require "medicating"). When the criteria for this particular "disorder" were tested, it was found to be impossible to distinguish between women with strong premenstrual symptoms, and those who were supposed to have this "disorder"; and even men gave answers that would satisfy a diagnosis of Premenstrual Dysphoric Disoder. And for this fictitious condition, the FDA approved the antidepressant Prozac (from Eli Lilly).[1]

In 2009 in the USA, the most sold drugs were anti-psychotics, with anti-depressants being the fourth best seller.[2] In 2012, The US Centres for Disease Control reported that 25% of all Americans had been diagnosed as having a mental illness.[3] And about 25% of the children in American summer camps were being medicated for mental problems.[4] Among those children who did not have a real medical condition before they were "medicated", it is known that 10% who take drugs for ADHD will develop bipolar disorder, caused by the drug.[5]

In 2010, the US Centres for Disease Control and Prevention reported that 9% of the adults they interviewed met the criteria for a diagnosis of depression.[6] The criteria were as commonplace as "poor appetite or overeating" combined with "having little interest or pleasure in doing things for more than half the days over the past two weeks".[7] With such definitions of depression (instigated by drug companies, or those they sponsor), it is not surprising that since anti-depressant drugs became available, the rate of diagnosed depression in the US has multiplied by 1,000.[8]

In the third edition of the DSM, a period of one year was considered normal for a person to suffer from bereavement. However, in the fifth edition, if you are now bereaved for more than two weeks, this is considered a mental condition (and you must be "medicated"). This has now become one of the normal states that is considered to be among the 374 mental conditions that a normal person needs "medication" for.[9]

In this situation, it is not surprising that 100% of the DSM panel members for "mood disorders" had financial ties to drug companies.[10]

Has psychiatry gone mad?

It seems that psychiatry has, itself, now gone mad. Normality has now become a mental condition that must be "medicated" for. This is in line with the drug industry policy of taking almost any drug (designed for any purpose), and reapplying it to any condition they can, by producing fraudulent trials and statistics to claim the drug improves these conditions, whether the condition is a real illness or not. It appears that it does not matter to the drug companies that their drugs are only doing harm to people and not improving their life in any way. The only guiding principle is profit, by any method (legal or otherwise), and at any cost to world health.

8. Drug companies create fictitious illnesses to boost profits

For example, the drug escitalopram is an anti-depressant produced by the Danish drug company Lundbeck. It is an SSRI drug (selective serotonin reuptake inhibitor). These drugs are controversial and there is much evidence of the great harm they do to people (p.63). Lundbeck sponsored a trial to claim that their SSRI anti-depressant, if taken by healthy menopausal women, could reduce the number of hot flushes per day from 10 to 9.[11] This is a tiny reduction, and even if the claim is true, the figure is an average and this tiny reduction would not be achieved in many women who took it. As shown on pages 79 to 99, there are many ways that drug companies routinely cheat to produce a trial that wrongly claims their drug has a benefit. But even if this trial were produced in good faith, and the analysis done honestly, it would be almost impossible to conduct such a trial in a truly blind or double blind way (SSRI's have conspicuous adverse effects, and most women on the trial who took the drug would have known they were taking it, rather than a placebo pill), and this bias is enough to produce a false positive outcome in favour of the drug.

Most doctors do not understand the issues related to drugs or drug trials, as explored in this book. In this instance, they would simply be aware that escitalopram (Cipralex, Lexapro, etc.) can be prescribed for menopausal hot flushes, so when faced with such a patient, many doctors would prescribe the drug. But SSRI's can have severe adverse effects. For example, a study found that people over 65 who take SSRI's are more likely to experience a fall than people who took older types of anti-depressants, or had no treatment at all.[12]

In other words, a healthy menopausal woman would be given this dangerous anti-depressant drug because she complained of hot flushes; and the only likely outcome would be that her hot flushes were not reduced; she had an increased risk of falling; and she would also experience the many other adverse effects that such drugs have. The only positive outcome would be that the drug company got richer, and the (also highly paid) doctor was able to get the woman out of his surgery to make his day easier.

The madness of psychiatry

SSRI's are widely used in psychiatry. Just before these drugs came on the market (in 1987), around 14,000 children in the USA were diagnosed as having a mental condition. But twenty years later, this number had increased to 500,000.[13] These figures suggest that just because this drug was now available (and drug company marketing claims it can be used for a wide range of psychiatric conditions), then psychiatrists (many sponsored in one way or another by drug companies[14]) tend to diagnose these conditions in children who would not previously have been diagnosed with having any condition.

There is controversy about drugs that affect the mind. It is considered that if these drugs are taken long term, then they are likely to cause the person to acquire the disease that the drug is supposed to have a positive effect on.[5] Another common adverse effect of these drugs is that they cause violence towards others, including murder. An analysis of adverse drug effects reported to the FDA over a five year period, found 1,937 cases of violence, and 387 of these were homicides.[15]

A drug widely used by psychiatrists

SSRI's are a notoriously dangerous drug. The first (Prozac) was introduced in 1987. No one knows why SSRI's have the effects they have.[16] In the UK these drugs were first promoted using false information provided by the drug regulator. It was wrongly claimed that depression was the result of a lack of the hormone serotonin in the brain.

The drug (a Selective Serotonin Reuptake Inhibitor) is supposed to increase the amount of serotonin in circulation. But whenever this type of approach is used to design drugs (which it is with most drugs), the "science" is incomplete and mainly misguided (Chapter 9). There is not even any reliable evidence that SSRI's combat depression. As with most trials that drug companies produce to promote their produces, the trials of SSRI's are flawed by bias.[17] And as with most drugs, the drug acts through the whole body, affecting all the organs and tissue; and most of its serious adverse effects cannot be explained (that is, it is not understood by the drug designers how their drug produces these effects).

One common adverse effect is on a person's sex life. In a study of this problem, it was found that 59% of patients (who all had a normal sex life before they took the drug) developed sexual problems, including decreased libido, delayed orgasm or ejaculation, no orgasm or ejaculation, sexual dysfunction, and yawning during orgasm.[18] But because this knowledge would be bad for drug sales, the drug companies claimed that only 5% (not 59%) of patients experience these sexual problems.[19]

What was so wonderful about Prozac?

The first SSRI was fluoxetine (better known as Prozac) and was produced by Eli Lilly. It was finally approved in 1988, after a long and arduous battle between Lilly and the drug regulators. In Germany and Sweden, the regulators (and even psychiatrists—who are not known for being shy of prescribing), considered the drug far too dangerous to approve;[19] and in the US, the FDA noted serious flaws in the trials of this drug that Lilly had conducted.[19] But Eli Lilly were facing the failure of their company if this drug was not approved.[20] They pressed their Swedish director, John Virapen, to do whatever it took to obtain approval for the drug in Sweden. Doctors were bribed to try out the drug on their patients before it was approved (known as a "seeding trial").[21] The independent expert who was going to examine the clinical trials was initially also against Prozac, but after a $20,000 bribe was paid, together with the promise of a large amount of research money for his department, the drug was approved.

In the registration application, deaths that had occurred during the trials were covered up. The original reports stated that "five had hallucinations and tried to commit suicide, which four of the test subjects succeeded in doing". This was changed to "Five of the other test subjects had miscellaneous effects." And approval in Germany was also achieved by using "unorthodox lobbying methods exercised on independent members of the regulatory authorities."[21]

After concealing the increased risk of suicide and violence associated with Prozac, Eli Lilly illegally promoted the drug for several non-approved ailments, including shyness, eating disorders and low self esteem.[19]

In 1990, Martin Teicher published a paper describing six patients who had become suicidal, reacting with intense and violent suicidal preoccupations while taking Prozac.[22] At the subsequent FDA hearings in 1991, Teicher's testimony was suppressed.

In 2002, documents came to light that revealed as far back as the 1980's Eli Lilly knew about the adverse effects of Prozac in relation to suicidal attempts and violence. The documents also revealed that Lily were keen to root out the word "suicide" from its database of adverse effects related to Prozac. It was directed by Lilly that when doctors reported to the company a suicide attempt on Prozac, this was to be coded as "overdose", and when it was reported that a patient had suicidal thoughts, this was to be coded as "depression".[23] In one of these documents, it was noted that in clinical trials, 38% of the patients who were given Prozac, reported "new activation". This is an extreme form of restlessness, which some patients describe as wanting to jump out of their skin, and it is associated with an increased risk of suicide.[19]

In 1989, one month after he was placed on Prozac, a man shot dead eight people and wounded another twelve, before killing himself.[24] At court, a jury ruled in Lilly's favour, which Lilly later used in marketing, claiming it had been "proven in a court of law… that Prozac is safe and effective." But it later transpired that Lilly had made a secret settlement with the plaintiffs during the trial. The judge changed the verdict from one in Lilly's favour, to "Dismissed as settled with prejudice," saying "Lilly sought to buy not just the verdict but the court's judgement as well."

Through the 1990's Lilly continued claiming publically that Prozac did not increase the risk or suicide or violence, while settling lawsuits out of court and seeking court orders to seal the documents, to keep the incriminating evidence hidden. But when a batch of these documents was leaked to the press, these revealed Lilly's campaign of disinformation about the harms of Prozac.[25]

8. Drug companies create fictitious illnesses to boost profits

In 1991, the FDA reviewed the safety of Prozac, but its panel members, several of whom had financial ties to Lilly, concluded that Prozac was safe. In a report to the FDA, Lilly excluded 76 of 97 cases of suicidality on Prozac that had been reported to them.[26, 27]

By 1997, Prozac was the fifth most prescribed drug in the USA, even though there had been hundreds of suicides reported while taking the drug.[28]

Internal documents from Lilly revealed that the company had known since 1978 that Prozac can produce in some people a strange, agitated state of mind that can trigger in them an unstoppable urge to commit suicide or murder.[29]

By 1999, the FDA had received reports of over 2,000 Prozac-associated suicides, and a quarter of the reports specifically referred to this agitated state of mind. However the FDA declined to require Lilly to place a warning about suicide on the drug's information leaflet.[30]

In 2004, Lilly conducted a clinical study of another of its SSRI's, duloxetine (Cymbalta), which they wanted to market for incontinence. A healthy 19-year-old college student volunteered to take part to help pay her college tuition. She was thoroughly screened to rule out depression or suicidal tendencies. After taking the drug, she committed suicide. This was concealed by Lilly. When researchers and the press started asking questions about the drug, the FDA declined to publish the data, claiming it was a trade secret belonging to Lilly.[26] After several freedom of information requests were filed to obtain the safety data on Cymbalta, the database was released and was found to contain 41 deaths and 13 suicides amongst patients taking Cymbalta. Missing from the database was any record of the college student and at least four other volunteers known to have committed suicide while taking Cymbalta. The FDA did later admit that when middle-aged women took this drug for incontinence, this doubled the rate of suicidal attempts amongst those women.

Impenetrable statistics are used to mislead

Despite all the clear evidence of cheating by drug companies to produce fraudulent trial results to promote their products, the false claims they make for their drugs are difficult for doctors and anyone else to unravel. Most doctors do not understand drugs, but statistics can be even more impenetrable. The following trials produced clear results that demonstrate the simple truth.

The real evidence is that antidepressants such as SSRIs, have little positive effect on most patients. In 2000, a four month trial of sertraline (or Zoloft; an SSRI antidepressant) on 156 patients with major depression was conducted. About half took the drug, and the other half merely exercised each day and took no drug. Six months later, 70% of the patients who merely exercised were no longer depressed, while 52% of the patients who took the drug were still depressed.[31] In other words, the trial showed that your health will improve far more if you simply conduct a normal life and take no pharmaceuticals.

In 2003, a similar trial was conducted. This time, the effect of sertraline on patients with a so-called "social phobia" was compared with the effects of not taking the drug but being gradually exposed to the phobia (in other words, simply returning to living a normal life). Initially, the improvement in both groups was similar, but six months later, the group who were exposed to the social situation they feared, continued to improve, whereas the group who took the drug, did not continue to improve.[32]

Glaxo concealed the addictiveness of its drug

In 1992, paroxetine, which is another SSRI (better known as Paxil, or Sereoxat) was first marketed by SmithKline Beecham, which later merged to become GlaxoSmithKline. In their original licence application, the company admitted that the drug led to withdrawal reactions in 30% of patients.[33] However, for the following ten years, the company claimed that the drug was not habit forming. Then, in 2001, the World Health Organization found that Paxil had the hardest withdrawal problems of any antidepressant drug. The International Federation of Pharmaceutical Manufacturers Associations found the company guilty of misleading the public about Paxil. And in 2003, Glaxo finally changed its prescribing instructions. It had originally claimed that the risk of withdrawal reactions was only 0.2%. It now admitted that the true figure was 25% (100 times more than they originally stated).[34]

Psychiatric propaganda that assists drug sales

Psychiatry is a big friend of drug companies. When patients are pushed into taking such drugs as SSRI antidepressants, and then try to stop, they are invariably misinformed that the withdrawal symptoms are, in fact, their original condition returning, therefore they must take the drug for life.

A common verse of drug company propaganda is related to the myth of chemical imbalances. The argument goes like this. Antidepressants are necessary to fix a chemical imbalance in someone's brain, therefore the person cannot stop taking the pill; the argument claims that such people are dependent on antidepressants in the same way that some diabetes patients are dependent on insulin injections.[35]

In relation to psychiatry, this is pure drug-company propaganda. But the example of diabetes patients being dependent on insulin injections, is also propaganda, this time from general mainstream healthcare. This is because diabetes can be simply cured with natural healing (p.117), and no insulin injections would then be needed at all. Instead the patient's pancreas and adrenal gland function is returned to normal with a simple treatment (that has been known about for over 2,000 years). Or the patient adopts a normal lifestyle, and the symptoms clear naturally.

9. An outsider's assessment of mainstream healthcare

From the previous chapters, many readers would naturally wonder why drug companies have resorted to behaving as they do now (with extensive use of fraud, and the concealing of the fatal harms of their products), and why mainstream healthcare has adopted such drug remedies as their main therapeutic tool.

The only effective healing discipline that has been portrayed in this book is traditional Chinese acupuncture. But historically Chinese herbal medicine has also been extremely effective, and uses the same diagnostic methods as acupuncture (to be able to tackle all the symptoms listed on pages 9 to 13). Herbal remedies are available today. But for this medicine to be used as a frontline healthcare system, the important distinction is that the herbal remedies should be prescribed by a practitioner of traditional Chinese medicine, who prepares the prescription for each individual patient.

Why were these powerful remedies not simply copied by drug companies?

Such herbal remedies may contain up to about fourteen different herbs. It is difficult to determine the biochemical characteristics of just a single herb, but when the mixture contains up to fourteen different herbs, the task of determining its characteristics becomes almost impossible.[1] And the current drug approval process does not accommodate undifferentiated mixtures of natural chemicals anyway.[2] Also any particular remedy would be mixed up for one particular patient; it could not legitimately be applied to all patients, to target a particular symptom—the remedy treats the overall person, not just a single symptom, just as traditional acupuncture does. Therefore these powerful herbal remedies could not be reproduced by the drug industry.

Why Use Natural Healing?

A notable exception to this is a highly effective malaria treatment, which is based on an ancient Chinese medicine herbal treatment. The main herb used was *Artemisia annua*. In 1972, a team from the China Academy of Chinese Medical Sciences identified the herb's active ingredient artemisinin,[3] which is now used to produce a successful malaria drug.

The current understanding of physiology and how the body's chemistry constantly varies to coordinate every aspect of our physiology, is limited. Only simple mechanisms are understood (similar to that described on p.33), and due to the current nature of biochemical engineering, the main option available in drug design is to try to block this simple chemistry (as described on pages 37-48). In general, with the current knowledge and technology, this is the only way that a centralized, mass-production-orientated drug industry can operate.

Given that this was the only avenue open to them, and mass produced remedies became the health industry's requirement, this is the direction that the drug industries and mainstream healthcare took.

But with most of the drugs that are now used, it was found that the understanding of how the body's overall chemistry works was inadequate. The drugs often did not even produce the intended outcome, and always produced a wide range of random adverse effects that had not been predicted by the drug's designers (which demonstrated that their knowledge was inadequate).

This was where the morality of big business took over. When regulation was required, by the drug companies trialling their drugs before approval, if these trials were done scientifically, the outcome was often simply a proof that the drug did not work. But by massaging the data and also using tricks to hide the worst of the harms (Chapters 5-8) a company could produce a fraudulent trial outcome that claimed the drug did work, and that its harms were within "acceptable" limits, even when the drug was dangerous, harmful to a person's health, and ineffective. This was not only a very lucrative practice, but some drug companies have found themselves facing closure if they did not cheat in these ways.[4] Extensive bribery was also used to ensure that any "regulation" was ineffective; and doctors were also bribed to use each drug company's products (Chapter 5). A drug trial is now nothing but drug company propaganda, produced for the sole purpose of generating profit, usually to the detriment of healthcare (Chapter 6).

This is now the mainstream healthcare approach that all developed countries use.

Why is this a problem?

Apart from the fact that very many healthy people are having their long-term health impeded by commonly used drugs, the biggest problem is that this approach is inept and cannot properly remedy fairly simple health conditions.

This limitation stems from the fact that today's knowledge of biochemistry does not provide a way to simply return an organ to normal function. The main device that drugs use so far is to chemically block the function of relatively superficial (and healthy) mechanisms.

When an organ malfunctions, this produces a whole range of possible symptoms (pp.9-13), but today's mainstream healthcare is usually not even aware that an organ is malfunctioning, and it only sees each of the resultant symptoms as a problem in its own right. Therefore it imagines that its crude intervention (in chemically blocking the function of a mechanism in the less-important tissue, which then prevents the symptom from manifesting) is somehow solving the problem.

For example, with over 2,000 years of consistent clinical results, Chinese medicine is aware that the underlying cause of most instances of hay fever and other allergies is poor function of the "kidneys"; and when the "kidney" function is corrected with acupuncture, the patient is cleared of all such allergies. This has also been my own clinical experience, with life-long sufferers suddenly being cleared of the condition, in what (to them) seems like a miraculous cure. But today's mainstream healthcare is unaware of such medical insights, and instead only uses antihistamines (p.182) to attempt to block the chemistry that enables the superficial symptoms to appear (itching nose and throat, red and sore eyes), but the underlying cause is left unchanged, to produce all the other symptoms it does (p.11), and to get progressively worse. And the patient must also suffer all the adverse effects of the drug. The same is true of asthma, IBS, stress-related symptoms, migraines and headaches, menstruation-related symptoms, and even many muscle and joint pains. In all these areas, traditional medicine can properly cure the condition by recognising which organ is malfunctioning to produce the symptoms, and returning that organ's function to normal.

This ineptitude caused yet another pandemic

In this respect, today's mainstream healthcare is totally inept. This was the real cause of the 2020 respiratory pandemic. This was a simple respiratory condition, related to a normal cold or flu, which feature a similar virus. The natural healing approach would be to return the lung and "kidney" functions to normal, which can be done within seconds with traditional acupuncture. Then, any patient who was struggling with the condition, would have been able to recover from it as they did from a normal cold (provided they were not taking drugs that prevented their organs from working normally). But instead, mainstream healthcare stood back, with doctors wringing their hands, saying "We can't treat this," and the whole world was brought to its knees by the ineptitude of mainstream healthcare. Whether this is a sufficient wakeup call, remains to be seen.

Other perspectives on the 2020 pandemic

It was found that the people who were unable to fight off this particular virus, were mainly those who had an underlying health condition. But another perspective on this which would not have occurred to medics, is that it was not the frailty of these people that made them victims, but it was the fact that they were routinely taking pharmaceuticals. These would prevent most of their main organs from functioning properly (p.58), and hence render them unable to fight off a variant of the common cold. Yet, people who were not taking such drugs, often did not even notice they had the virus, or could shake it off like a mild cold or flu, as normal. In other words, their immunity worked normally, because it was not impeded by the chemical blocking of their main organ functions.

And another perspective is this. In my own acupuncture practice I had been noticing for years that with each bout of seasonal colds or flu,

9. An outsider's assessment of mainstream healthcare

the symptoms that people experienced were getting more and more unusual. One possible explanation for this is as follows. In recent decades, for the first time in evolution, a large portion of farm animals, pets and humans had the normal function of their organs and tissue impeded with prescription drugs (p.58). This means that their bodies now worked differently from the way they had worked for millions of years. And perhaps pathogens were (in effect) taking advantage of this situation. Hence people were experiencing slightly modified symptoms with a common cold or flu. If this is the explanation for the new strains, such as those that first appeared in 2019 and the later variants, then the drug industry had accidentally engineered this situation, and all similar pandemics that may arise in the near future—until the world bans the ridiculous policy of chemically blocking the normal function of our bodily organs and tissue. In other words, bans the majority of prescription drugs currently used.

By default, the focus turned to combating pathogens
This ineptitude is perhaps also the reason why mainstream healthcare has become obsessed with doing battle with pathogens, such as bacteria and viruses. In the absence of being able to return the main organs to normal function, so that the body's own defences deal with pathogens, just as they had always done; mainstream healthcare has defaulted to the position of instead attempting to kill the pathogens—simply because it cannot perform normal healing.

In fairness, perhaps it became obsessed with this simply because it could imagine how to perform this task, with the limited knowledge available to them. And because it *could* do battle with pathogens, this, by default, became the main focus of this medical religion (one of its central tenets). But there are many scientists who think even this standard "germ theory" is untrue, which is covered starting on page 140.

Even if unintentionally, the preaching of this tenet now forms a central part of the endless scaremongering that is so familiar from mainstream healthcare (keeping the faithful in check). The mantra goes something like, "It is the virus or bacteria that is the problem; we must kill those," and they instil into people a fear of breathing the very air that keeps them alive.

Notably, during this pandemic which had brought the world to its knees, and which was the product of the ineptitude of the mainstream medical religion, the propaganda arm of that religion arranged for all books or material relating the objective facts about vaccination to be banned from sale. This ban was enacted by the likes of Amazon, and reinforced by politicians and mainstream medical authorities.[5] Like any powerful religion, they only permit the promotion of their own message and take whatever steps they can to silence the opposition. Any opposing text is labelled as "misinformation". This is understandable, since this is how most commercial, political, and publicity organizations conduct themselves. But when the subject matter is world health, it is a dangerous position when such a damaging, misguided medical religion gains a monopoly on thought.

Chemical blocking of normal, healthy function

This inability to correct organ malfunctions, or to even be able to detect such malfunctions, has led mainstream healthcare to use this same crude, inept approach in many common areas of healthcare.

This approach is used in asthma. Chinese medicine knew over 2,000 years ago that the underlying cause of most cases of asthma is a weakness in the "kidney" function; and treating the "kidneys" with acupuncture immediately clears the breathing difficulty. Consistent clinical results have been obtained over all this time, and I have seen this mechanism in action many times with my own patients. Yet, because today's physiology has yet to discover this relationship between the "kidneys" and the lungs' ability to breathe in, mainstream healthcare is unaware of the underlying cause of this type of asthma. Instead, drugs are used to block the normal function of the airways in the lungs. This is similar to the approach used with blood-pressure issues, where the normal function of the muscles surrounding the blood vessels is chemically blocked, so that the muscles expand. The airways in the lungs also have smooth muscle surrounding them, which performs a vital function during respiration. In asthmatic patients, these muscles

9. An outsider's assessment of mainstream healthcare

seem to increase in mass and contraction. Though today's physiology does not know why this happens,[6] the drug-based response to asthma is to chemically block this smooth muscle from working, so that it relaxes, thus expanding the airways and making it easier to breathe, in the short term. But this does not in any way tackle the cause of the problem, which is left untreated; and the danger is that by chemically blocking the airway smooth muscle from working, this may seriously weaken the lungs' normal function in the long term. In contrast, traditional acupuncture treats the underlying cause, which is in the "kidney" function, and this immediately corrects any problem in the airway smooth muscle of the lungs.

With most of the other symptoms produced by organ malfunction (as listed on pages 9 to 13), instead of correcting the genuine problem in the organ, the distal symptom is imagined to be a separate problem; and a normal, healthy function in the distal tissue is chemically blocked from working, to attempt to prevent this distal symptom from appearing. But because such drugs act systemically, this also inhibits functions in all the main organs (p.58), which then produces the unpredicted adverse effects of these drugs; and thereby does untold damage to the person's long-term health. And when this approach then produces other symptoms in reaction to the drug, these are imagined to be new, separate problems, and a further drug is added to chemically block another aspect of the body that was functioning normally; and the person's health continues its decline.

Another approach, when mainstream healthcare has noticed that an organ is malfunctioning but they cannot correct the malfunction, is to attempt to perform the organ's role themselves, as far as they can understand it. This approach is used with diabetes. Our pancreas is the main digestive organ; amongst many other tasks, it produces insulin, which plays a role in enabling the body to use the glucose from our diet. When it is noticed that the pancreas' production of insulin is not adequate, instead of correcting the function, insulin is artificially injected into the patient, to take the place of this aspect of the pancreas function. From the natural healing perspective, doing this is yet another way of blocking the organ from ever returning to normal function; whereas in natural healing, the pancreas function is simply returned to normal, and the symptoms clear.

Within mainstream healthcare, the practice of chemically blocking normal, healthy function is considered to be "medicine". And the fact that these drug remedies harm the patient's health (with adverse effects) is accepted as normal.

Today's medical religion

It is appropriate to label this system a medical religion. Among its central tenets are the claims that it is scientific and evidence-based. It is neither. The fraud related to drug trials documented in this book alone (chapters 5-8) is an abandonment of all scientific principles. But even putting aside this routine fraud, the approach of drug designers cannot be considered scientific. It is common to take a drug that chemically blocks a particular mechanism, and blindly try this on patients who have a condition totally different to that the drug was initially designed for, just to see if (by chance) it produces any effect on their unrelated condition. This is nothing less than randomly blocking the body's chemistry in the hope that the harmful effects are not too bad (the drug can be "tolerated", as they say), and that there is some positive outcome in a small percent of people.

This is not scientific. It is taking random stabs in the dark. And the fact that most drugs produce unpredicted harmful effects, is itself a demonstration that they are not scientifically designed. If they were, there would not be any unpredicted effects. These effects occur because the models used to design drugs are inadequate (in other words, the biochemical engineers do not fully understand the complex chemistry of the body); hence the models could not predict the outcome. And as shown in chapters 6 and 7, this practice usually involves the drug company then performing a pseudo trial, and fraudulently manipulating the data (and also often hiding evidence of the worst harmful effects), to obtain a fake trial outcome that claims to "prove" the drug is effective.

This is not medicine at all. And it certainly is not science. When the evidence has to be faked, the practice also cannot legitimately be claimed to be evidence based.

A catch-phrase (or further tenet of this religion) that is frequently heard is "The benefits of a drug outweigh its harm." But this cannot be properly determined. They are usually oblivious of which organ functions are impeded by the drug (p.58) and therefore what the long-term effects of the drug are. They do not know the full effects of the harm, so they cannot make the calculation.

The real calculation should be, is it better to do nothing (p.108), or go ahead and chemically block a person's organ functions in a random way? The properly considered answer to this would always be that it is better to do nothing, because the drug intervention would be ruling out the possibility that the person's main organs would ever be able to function normally.

Healthcare that really is scientific

In contrast, the approach adopted by Chinese medicine is far more scientific. It determines which organ is producing the symptom, confirms this with several different, reliable diagnostic tests, then specifically treats the one target organ to return it to normal function; and this result is then confirmed by reusing any of the diagnostic tests, and by the fact that the symptoms clear, reliably, century after century. This is totally scientific, and genuinely evidence based; and involves no fraud, sleight of hand, nor greed or profit, and puts today's mainstream healthcare to shame.

I have mentioned the tendency in mainstream healthcare to theorize about how the body works on the chemical level, then attempt to produce a treatment by impeding this chemistry. The reason why this produces so much harm to the patient is that the knowledge is incomplete.

In ancient China, the intellectuals also theorized about how the body works. In effect, those theories were mostly metaphorical and were not literally true.[7] But the important difference from today's approach, is that Chinese acupuncture treatment does not rely on those ancient, untrue theories. The system was discovered through practical observations, which were all factual. And the theorizing came later, by intellectuals who wanted to try to explain what was happening in the body. These can be viewed as charming, poetic ideas but are not really related to what happens in the body during an acupuncture treatment. If instead, Chinese medicine had attempted to produce a treatment by directly manipulating these theorized substances and mechanisms, their treatments would have been as unsuccessful and as damaging to health as today's drug-based approach is. But fortunately, no part of traditional acupuncture treatment relies on those ancient theories, which is why it is so successful.

There is no doubt that the pharmaceutical industry is broken. It is corrupt and profit driven, at the expense of healthcare. But this is not the problem with mainstream healthcare. The problem is that this particular drug-based approach is fundamentally flawed from its conception. And that's the reason why most of the drug industry's products don't work.

But how could such an all-pervasive practice be abandoned?

It is true that the whole of the mainstream medical industry relies on this approach, from the training of doctors upwards, so it is difficult to imagine the complete abandonment of this approach, since so much state-sponsored infrastructure is now built around it. But it is just this situation that keeps such damaging and corrupt practices in place, ensuring that mainstream healthcare remains detrimental to world health. And the other thing that keeps this system intact is that the human body can endure all the ills done to it by this healthcare system and still survive—even if in bad health.

There is no quick fix. The system is fundamentally flawed, and unravelling all the died-in-the-wool misguided thinking is too huge a task. The only realistic solution is for enough people to recognise mainstream healthcare for what it is, and to turn to natural healing. People-power seems to be the only way that such a transformation could take place to then enable the modern world to enjoy real healthcare.

9. An outsider's assessment of mainstream healthcare

An occasional criticism of natural healing, by medics, is that it is placebo. But placebo does not exist; it is yet one more fraudulent notion invented by drug companies to attempt to justify their ineffective and harmful remedies (p.79); and medics only reach for this label because they do not understand real healing. It is beyond their training or imaginations.

It is disappointing that humanity has been duped into adopting such a practice for its mainstream healthcare when a sophisticated, powerful healing system with over 2,000 years of consistent clinical results, is widely known about and still practised. The solution to today's healthcare problems is hidden in plain sight.

10. Do vaccines work?

What is vaccination? The theory is that if an attenuated virus related to a disease is injected directly into a healthy person's blood, their immune system will form antibodies to that disease but without them developing the disease, which will provide them with immunity to the disease in future.

What are the facts?

There is a dramatic contrast between the historical facts related to vaccination and the claims of medical authorities. It is a frequent claim that vaccines were responsible for "eradicating" diseases such as polio, but this is simply not true. For example, the incidence and severity of whooping cough (pertussis) had already begun to dramatically decline long before the pertussis vaccine was introduced.[1] And the same is true of diphtheria, tetanus, TB, cholera, typhus, typhoid, which all began to disappear toward the end of the Nineteenth Century,[2] largely in response to improvements in public health and sanitation,[3,4] but in any case long before antibiotics or vaccines. It is also recorded that nearly 90% of the total decline in mortality for scarlet fever, diphtheria, whooping cough, and measles between 1860 and 1965 occurred before the introduction of antibiotics and widespread immunization.[5]

The great microbiologist René Dubos observed that microbial diseases have their own natural history, independent of drugs and vaccines, in which asymptomatic infection and symbiosis are much more common than overt disease. He said "Animals and plants, as well as men, can live peacefully with their most notorious microbial enemies. The world is obsessed by the fact that poliomyelitis can kill and maim several thousand unfortunate victims every year. But more extraordinary is the fact that millions upon millions of young people become infected by polio viruses, yet suffer no harm from the infection… Infection can occur without producing disease."[6]

What effect do vaccines have?

When a vaccine produces antibodies to a particular disease, the overall effect on a person's immunity to that disease appears to be different to the effect that results when a person contracts a disease naturally and recovers from it. The evidence is that artificially invoked antibodies do not have the same effect of providing the person with immunity. This is suggested by the fact that the corresponding diseases have continued to break out, even in highly immunized populations.

For example, in a 1977 British outbreak of whooping cough, even fully-immunized children contracted the disease in large numbers, and their rates of serious complications and death were not reduced significantly.[7]

In a 1969 outbreak of diphtheria in Chicago, the Board of Health reported that 25% of the cases had been fully immunized; another 12% had received one or more doses and serologically were fully "immune;" and another 18% had been partly immunized, according to the same criteria.[8]

In 1977, 34 new cases of measles were reported on the UCLA campus, among a population that was supposedly 91% immune, according to careful serological testing.[9]

The facts about the polio vaccine

That vaccines "eradicated" polio, is a message that has been repeated so many times by medical authorities that it has become a staple of vaccine folklore in the minds of the media and public. But is there any truth behind this claim?

According to US medical statistics, polio decreased from 18,000 cases in 1954, to fewer than 20 in 1973-78. This remarkable claim was investigated. In a 1978 congressional hearing,[10] Dr Bernard Greenburg reported that not only did the incidence of polio increase substantially after the compulsory mass vaccination program began, but that statistics were manipulated to give the opposite impression.

In 1957, the North Carolina Health Dept claimed that polio decreased in the state from 1953 to 1957, after public vaccination. However, Dr Fred Clenner of North Carolina pointed out that it wasn't until 1955 that a single person in the state received the polio vaccine. And the numbers vaccinated were on a very limited bases, since the vaccine was causing so many cases of polio. It wasn't until 1956 that polio vaccinations became widespread in North Carolina. Therefore, the 61% drop in polio was credited to the Salk vaccine when it had not even been used in the state. And in 1957, when mass vaccination began, polio again increased.

There were several other ways the authorities used to manipulate the data to attempt to demonstrate that the vaccine worked. One way was that after mass vaccination was introduced, the definition of a polio epidemic was changed. Previously, there only needed to be 20 cases in 100,000 of the population, and an epidemic was declared. But after the vaccination was introduced, they raised the definition to 100 cases in 100,000 of the population. This meant that even if the new vaccine produced a 75% increase in the number of polio cases, an epidemic was still not declared. Therefore it could be claimed that the vaccine had cleared an epidemic, no matter how many extra cases of polio the vaccine had in fact caused.

Another method used was to change the criteria for diagnosing polio. Before mass vaccination, for a patient to be diagnosed as having paralytic poliomyelitis (polio), the patient only needed to have paralytic symptoms for 1 day (24 hours). After the vaccine, this was increased to 60 days. This made it more or less impossible for a doctor to diagnose polio. Many people still presented with polio, but now it had to be called something else. This was most often "spinal meningitis". Both these supposedly different diseases have essentially identical symptoms. Therefore, after the polio vaccination was introduced, there appeared an epidemic of "spinal meningitis" (in other words, a new epidemic of polio).

These simple devices allowed health authorities to make the false claim that the polio vaccination had eradicated polio. Despite this attempt at a medical cover-up, polio increases were still reported in many US states. The yearly figures for some states, before and after the polio vaccine were:
- Tennessee: 119 cases before; 386 cases after vaccination;

- Ohio: 17 cases before; 52 after;

- Connecticut: 45 cases before; 123 after;

- North Carolina: 78 cases before; 313 after vaccination.[11]

The medical propaganda is widely believed, since it tends to be the only source of information. Its usual claim is that in the United States (for example), there was one big polio epidemic in the 1940's, and this dreadful disease was eradicated by Jonas Salk's vaccine. But the truth is that polio had always occurred in cycles. In the US, there was an epidemic in the 1910's and in the 1930's, and both these epidemics cleared naturally. This was because there was no polio vaccine keeping the disease alive in the population. In Europe, polio disappeared naturally in the 1940's and 1950's, without vaccines. It had also virtually disappeared in the US, before the vaccination program began, which then only had the opposite effect. And this effect was confirmed by Salk himself (the vaccine's developer) who stated that in the US, between 1966 and 1976, two thirds of the cases of polio were caused by his vaccine.[12]

Between 1955 and 1963, the polio vaccine was produced in monkey kidney cell cultures, which harboured Simian Virus 40 (SV40), which is now known to cause cancer in humans. In 1960, it was discovered that SV40 contaminated up to 30% of the poliovirus vaccines in the US. During this period, approximately 90% of children and 60% of adults in the US were inoculated for polio and possibly exposed to this cancer-causing SV40.[13]

In 2003, in the American Journal of Medicine, RA Vilchez stated: "SV40 (a monkey virus found in polio vaccines) is associated significantly with brain tumours, bone cancers, malignant mesothelioma, and non-Hodgkins lymphoma."

History of the small pox vaccine

As far back as 1895, a Dr Charles Craten, writing in the Encylopedia Britannica, wrote of his research into the effects of the small pox vaccination, and noted many instances of the vaccine causing syphilis in children. In 1899, Sir Alfred Russel Wallace, compiled pages of data from the available records of his time and concluded that the small pox vaccination was a complete fraud, which caused more small pox than it cured; and that enforced vaccination was a crime.

The esteemed author George Bernard Shaw wrote that during the small pox epidemic at the turn of the century, the authorities maintained the statistical credit of vaccines by misdiagnosing all the vaccinated cases of small pox as "pustular exema," amongst other things. They would call such cases anything but small pox, because the child was previously vaccinated for small pox, so it could not be admitted that they had contracted small pox. The small pox vaccine was eventually discontinued due to the amount of cases of small pox caused by the vaccine.

Australia and New Zealand were practically unvaccinated at the time, and were more free from small pox than any other country. The most vaccinated nations were Italy, the Philippines, Mexico, and India. And all these nations were scourged with small pox. After the US-led vaccine program in the Philippines, they experienced the largest epidemic of small pox to ever hit their country. 162,000 cases and 71,000 deaths were reported in vaccinated people. The experience in Japan was similar. By 1892, their records showed 165,000 cases with over 29,000 deaths in vaccinated people. Whereas in Australia, where there was no compulsory small pox vaccinations, there were only 3 deaths in 15 years.[14]

In 1999, a medical researcher, Glen Dettman, stated: "Smallpox would never have been the problem it was if the smallpox vaccine was not invented and promoted. In populations where there was no vaccine, there was no smallpox."

The measles vaccine

There is a similar picture with measles. The disease began to decline around 1900, and it sharply declined (by about 90%) from 1948 to 1958. The first measles vaccine was licensed in 1963, but was not in wide use until 1967, when the disease had already declined naturally. However, the medical authorities wrongly claim that it was the measles vaccine that "eradicated" the disease.

In 1986, a Morbidity and Mortality Report found that 80% of measles outbreaks occurred in vaccinated populations.

In 1987, a study in the Journal of Epidemiology found that out of 137 cases of childhood measles studies, 99% were vaccinated for measles.

In 1990, a New Zealand study found that MMR vaccination programs this year created a tremendous outbreak of spinal meningitis.

In 2000, a study in the Journal of Epidemiology found that the Brazilian meningitis outbreak was created by MMR vaccination programs.

The whooping cough vaccine

Between 1850 and 1950, the US child population had increased enormously. And during this time, incidence of death from whooping cough decreased from over 1,000 per million to less than 10 per million, which all occurred prior to any mass vaccination programs. The same was true for measles, diphtheria, scarlet fever and TB.[15]

After the start of vaccination programs in the UK, it was found that over 45% of whooping cough cases occurred in fully vaccinated children. In 1981 in Sweden and the UK, whooping cough vaccination was decreased, and the whooping-cough death rates dropped dramatically.[16]

As well as not being effective, the pertussis (whooping cough) vaccine carries a high risk of known adverse effects. Its ability to damage the Central Nervous System, for example, became clear when Dr. Gordon Stewart and his colleagues reported the high incidence of encephalopathy and severe convulsive disorders in British children that were traceable to the vaccine.[17]

A 1988 study in the Journal of the American Medical Association found that there is substantial under reporting of whooping cough (pertussis) in the United States; and that whooping cough occurs at a far greater rate now than before the introduction of the vaccine.

In 1989, a Morbidity and Mortality Report found that whooping cough (pertussis) outbreaks occurred in 100% vaccinated populations.

In 1998, a study published in the Journal of the American Medical Association found that 98% of children with whooping cough (pertussis) were vaccinated for the disease.

In 2000, a Danish study found that the increase in whooping cough (pertussis) incidence is higher amongst vaccinated populations than it is in non-vaccinated populations of all ages.

The rabies vaccine

Louis Pasteur produced a rabies vaccine, but in France, more people died from his rabies vaccine than ever died of rabies. And France's Academy of Medicine found that "Pasteur's rabies vaccinations may be followed as much as 20 years later with a rare form of psychosis". In all countries where Pasteur's rabies vaccine was used, the number of deaths from rabies actually increased, rather than diminished. His vaccine was also given to King Alexander of Greece, after he was bitten by a monkey, and the king died of the vaccine within one week. Pasteur also produced an anthrax vaccine which was administered in Russia to 4,500 sheep, and 3,600 of them died almost immediately.

The theory of vaccination

All the above evidence suggests that vaccines do not, in fact, provide immunity to a particular disease. They may invoke the production of antibodies to that disease, but it is clear from the evidence that this does not then provide the person with immunity. Why is this?

How does our immunity respond to a disease?

Suppose a normal, healthy person contracts measles. How does their immunity cope with this? According to current physiology knowledge, once the virus is inhaled by a susceptible individual, it undergoes a prolonged period of multiplication, at progressively "deeper" levels of the body; beginning in the tonsils, and progressing (after several days) to the blood, spleen, thymus, and the bone marrow, which are the main "organs" of the immune system. This is known as the incubation period, which lasts from 10 to 14 days. Throughout this time, the person usually feels well and experiences few or no symptoms. By the time the first symptoms of measles appear, circulating antibodies are already detectable in the blood, and when the symptoms are at their most severe, this coincides with the peak of the antibody response.

An important natural-healing concept is that this type of infectious "illness" (considering all its symptoms together: the swelling, soreness, fever, coughing, and outpourings) is simply the body's (the immune system's) attempt to clear the virus from itself. This process of succumbing to and recovering from an acute illness like the measles involves the mobilization of many aspects of the immune system as a whole (much of it known but some not fully understood), of which the production of circulating antibodies is only one part.

In contrast, a vaccine focuses on only the antibody-production aspect of this whole immune response. It manages to produce antibodies, but without engaging every element of the immune response (all the known and unknown elements).

By injecting directly into the blood a modified measles virus, aspects of the immune system are "tricked" into producing antibodies. But this antibody response occurs as an isolated technical feat, without any overt illness to recover from. By focusing on this single aspect of immunity (antibody production), artificial immunization uses this to stand as a substitute for the whole immune response, in much the same way as elevated blood pressure is responded to by chemically blocking healthy systems in the body. This is accepted as a valid substitute for the healing of the underlying condition that led to the raised blood pressure (Chapter 3). This type of trickery does not benefit the person. In the case of blood-pressure issues, the underlying health problem is not addressed, and is usually not even known.

With vaccination, it is clear from the evidence that this trick does not work, because immunized people often contract the disease the vaccine is supposed to protect them from. And there is no evidence that vaccination has ever "eradicated" a disease; and plenty of evidence that it has increased the incidence of the diseases it has targeted.

This failure to work as theorized may be due to the fact that vaccination does not invoke the full, normal immune response and the process of recovering from this; in other words, becoming ill naturally and recovering from this. And because this full, normal process has not happened, the person has not acquired immunity to that particular disease.

As well as this failure to provide immunity, vaccines often create unusual new diseases, and also leave the person with the "seeds" of serious chronic disease lurking within their own cells.

Vaccines can produce atypical diseases

Vaccines do not only produce mild copies of the original disease; they also commonly produce a variety of symptoms of their own, which in some cases may be more serious than the symptoms of the target disease and harder to clear.

In a 1980 outbreak of mumps in supposedly immune schoolchildren, several developed atypical symptoms, such as anorexia, vomiting, and rashes, but with no swelling of the salivary glands (which is typical in mumps), and hence could not be diagnosed without extensive serological testing.[18] The syndrome of "atypical measles" can be equally difficult to diagnose, even when it is suspected.[19] And in some cases, atypical measles can be much more severe than the regular kind, with pneumonia, small red spots, swelling, and severe pain.[20]

How might vaccines cause autoimmune conditions?

It has long been known that live viruses are capable of surviving for years within host cells in a latent form, without necessarily provoking acute disease, simply by attaching their own genetic material as an episome, or extra particle, to the genome of the host cell and replicating along with it.[21] Latent viruses of this type have been implicated in chronic disease, such as herpes simplex; shingles; warts; kuru;[†] Creutzfeldt-Jakob disease; Guillain-Barré syndrome; subacute scleros-

---

[†] Kuru is usually caused by an infectious protein found in contaminated human brain tissue. It was previously found in people from New Guinea who ate the brains of dead people as part of a funeral ritual.

ing panencephalitis (SSPE), a rare complication of measles;[22] and also tumors, both benign and malignant.[23]

In all of these varieties, the latent virus survives as a foreign element within the cell, and because the virus is now permanently incorporated within the genetic material of the cell, when the immune system continues to make antibodies against it, these antibodies must now be directed against the cell itself.

Although it can seem inexplicable why a person's immune system should suddenly start attacking and destroying the person's own tissues, this phenomenon makes sense when considering that the immune system is merely attempting to destroy chronically infected cells to try to eliminate these foreign antigens persisting within the person's cells.

In 1976, Prof. Robert Simpson of Rutgers stated, "Immunization programs against flu, measles, mumps, polio, and so forth, may actually be seeding humans with RNA to form latent proviruses in cells throughout the body. These could be molecules in search of diseases: when activated under proper conditions, they could cause a variety of diseases, including rheumatoid arthritis, multiple sclerosis, systemic lupus erythematosus, Parkinson's disease, and perhaps cancer."[24]

Are antibodies the full story?

Putting aside the distinction between having artificially invoked antibodies or naturally invoked antibodies, the role that antibodies play in immunity is not fully understood anyway, and not all scientists accept the standard explanation.

There is a disorder called *agammaglobulinemia*, which some children are born with, which means that they are unable to produce antibodies. Some parents, on advice from doctors, place their child in a "bubble", so that they are not exposed to "germs". But many children with this disorder lead normal lives, and they are still able to recover spontaneously from diseases such as measles and other diseases, just as other children do. This, despite the fact that they cannot produce antibodies.[25]

However, the idea that "antibodies protect against disease" is a cardinal tenet for drug-company sponsored healthcare; and any study or evidence that disproves this tenet is rejected as "faulty". This happened in a 1950 study (the *British Medical Research Council* Report #272), which found that there was no correlation between diphtheria antibody counts in the blood and whether or not a person had diphtheria or had been exposed to it. Some such people had high counts, some had minimal counts. The study was terminated and declared a failure, since it suggested that the central theory on the role of antibodies in disease was untrue. However, it pointed to the simple fact that you do not necessarily need antibodies to recover from a disease.

Along with the constant reciting of such (religious) tenets, they are also used effectively to instigate much scaremongering.

The AIDS epidemic and HIV

This condition existed long before the term "AIDS" was coined in 1982. The condition was previously called *leukocytopenia*, meaning a decreased number of white blood cells, and hence, poor immunity. But in 1982, this term was changed to "AIDS" by America's Centres for Disease Control and Prevention, for the purposes of a press conference.

In the early 1990's, Dr Peter Duesberg, a prestigious university professor and viral researcher had published research that unequivocally found no connection between the HIV virus and AIDS.[26] This was born out in practice. When an autopsy of an AIDS victim was carried out, it was rare to find HIV. And there are thousands of medically diagnosed AIDS cases that had never tested positive for HIV.

On the other hand, there is a contradiction in the usual medical tenet and theories on this topic. If you test positive for HIV, then according to those tenets, surely this is a good thing, because the HIV antibody will protect you from getting AIDS. Therefore there should be no need to damage your immunity by taking toxic drugs.

An alternative perspective is that the presence of the HIV antibody in a person's blood does not indicate any particular disease, but more indicates that the person's blood is in the process of being clensed of the normal toxins that exist in most people's blood. But if the presence of HIV is detected, this wrongly leads to a diagnosis, and the person often takes extremely toxic drugs, such as AZT and/or other terri-

Why Use Natural Healing?

ble antiviral drugs, which would eventually harm the person's immunity and cause symptoms of AIDS. But since another key medical tenet goes "No drugs or vaccines could possibly be harmful, or cause disease or death," the wrong conclusion was that it is HIV that leads to AIDS.[27]

In a study conducted by the Concord Institute, an independent American research organization, it was found that 51% of the people using AZT develop lymphatic cancer. And in the AZT product information, among the adverse effects of the drug are many of the symptoms of AIDS.

In contrast, when people have been genuinely diagnosed with AIDS (or, to remove the scaremongering factor embodied in the term "AIDS", we could call it "diminished white blood cells"), when such people refuse all drugs, prescribed and otherwise, and clean up their lifestyle, including diet and exercise, the vast majority make a full recovery. If they also use natural healing to aid this detoxification process and speed up recovery, this can only help.[28]

However, Duesberg was ostracized for daring to question one of these cardinal medical tenets (that the presence of antibodies cannot confirm a diagnosis of disease, nor insure protection from it). Many of his colleagues went on record to say that his research was correct, but few lacked the courage to publicly support him, for fear of losing their own funding (understandably, no drug company could be expected to support any person or idea that threatened the very existence of the drug companies).

Dr Walter Gilbert, a Nobel prize winner in microbiology, stated "The major thing that concerns me by calling HIV the cause of AIDS is that we do not have a proof of causation."

Dr Joseph Sonnebend, a private AIDS researcher and clinition, stated "It is most definitely not a fact that HIV causes AIDS. That is a conjecture, and not an established fact."

Dr Robert Root-Bernstein, a physiologist at Michigan State University, commented that AIDS patients are given a multitude of immune-suppressant agents, and said "The logic of the war on AIDS is seriously flawed."

Dr Root-Bernstein also stated "Medical records show that HIV was in the blood stream of some patients, and that it infected some of their cells, and they developed antibodies to it, and that at a later time, HIV could no longer be found in them. In some cases, these people even lost their antibodies to HIV, and all have remained perfectly healthy."

Dr Peter Duesberg, a pioneering virologist at the University of California at Berkley, stated "There is no proof that HIV causes AIDS. In addition, I am familiar with retroviruses, how they behave and what they do, and on those counts I am confident enough that HIV, no matter how, couldn't possible cause AIDS."

So, how did the "AIDS" epidemic begin?

The most likely account is as follows. At the New York Blood Centre, a very experimental hepatitis B vaccine program was conducted in New York City, Chicago and San Francisco. All major papers in these cities ran ads for gay men to try the new vaccine in 1971 and 1972. And about ten years later, the major outbreaks of AIDS began in these cities. In other words, the vaccine was so toxic that it eventually destroyed the white blood cells, greatly damaging the immune system of the people it was designed to protect, producing the symptoms of AIDS.

In people who have an unhealthy lifestyle, including taking recreational drugs, their blood would ordinarily be fairly toxic (all people's blood has some level of toxicity, which is what the immune system is intended to clear). Hence HIV antibodies would be present in most such people, which does not provide a diagnosis of any sort. But during the height of the scaremongering around AIDS, any healthy person found to have the HIV antibody would have been persuaded to take further, extremely toxic drugs, which would have only compromised their immunity even further, eventually producing the symptoms of AIDS. In this scenario, the whole AIDS epidemic was medically induced, and medically perpetuated (by "medically", I mean the healthcare that is sponsored by drug companies).

The other toxic aspect of vaccines

Apart from frequently causing the disease they are supposed to protect against, and inducing autoimmune conditions, vaccines have also been linked to many other serious harms. What might explain this?

A vaccine is made up of an unnaturally large protein that contains many toxic substances. Apart from the material extracted from infected animals, they also typically contain substances like mercury (a potent neurotoxin), formaldehyde (a carcinogen), aluminium phosphate (which has been linked to nervous system breakdown), thimerosal (derived from mercury, and also neurotoxic), neomycin (suppresses immune system), ammonium sulphate (poisonous to the digestive organs, liver and nerves), and so on.

Normally, such a large protein would not be present in our blood. All proteins are broken down by our digestion, into amino acids. But with vaccines, this unusually large and toxic protein is injected directly into our blood. Such toxins, if inhaled or eaten, would usually be destroyed by our normal defences. But these defences are bypassed.

Once in our blood, such a large protein (which should not be there) may travel to our brain, which is one possible explanation for the brain and neurological damage that sometimes occurs after vaccination. Also, once a large protein is in the blood, it cannot be digested, and slowly decomposes, releasing its toxic contents.

In 1990, Harris Coulter, Ph.D, of the Centre for Empirical Medicine, stated that "15% to 20% of American school children are considered learning disabled with minimal brain damaged directly caused by vaccines."

The leaflet for a DPT (diphtheria, pertussis—or, whooping cough—and tetanus) vaccine states that these possible adverse effects have been associated with the vaccine.[29] But with the more serious conditions, the information usually states that the condition occurred after receiving the vaccine but that there is no proof that the vaccine caused the condition (in typical lawyer-speak):

- Collapse
- Prolonged prostration and shock like state

- Screaming or inconsolable crying
- Convulsions
- Unconsciousness
- Guillain-Barré syndrome (full body paralysis)
- Brachial neuritis (nerve damage)
- SIDS (Sudden infant death syndrome)
- Death due to serious infection

In 1982, a US TV show (called "DPT, vaccine routlette") described studies that confirmed the brain damage caused by this vaccine. After people became afraid to receive the vaccine, the AMA responded by claiming that the respective diseases were now rapidly climbing. A Dr Anthony Morris from the FDA visited Maryland and Wisconsin to verify these AMA claims of increased disease rates. However, he found that in Maryland only five of the 41 cases that were reported as diphtheria were confirmed. And all five of these children had actually been vaccinated with DPT. In Wisconsin, only 16 of the 43 reported cases of diphtheria were confirmed, and 14 of these confirmed cases had contracted the disease after being vaccinated.[30]

Dr Robert S. Mendelsohn, a famous American paediatrician and anti-vaccinationist, portrayed doctors as powerful priests of a primitive religion, with dishonesty as its central ethic. He stated "There is no convincing scientific evidence that mass vaccination programs can be credited with eliminating any childhood disease. I urge you to reject all vaccinations for your child." He also held that the methods of modern medicine were often more dangerous than the diseases they were designed to diagnose and treat.[31]

Sudden Infant Death Syndrome

Before mass vaccination programs began in the 1950's, "Crib death" was extremely rare. It only started to increase from the 1950's. Many routine vaccines are now given to young infants and even babies. In 1975, in response to the Sudden Infant Death Syndrome (SIDS) phenomenon, Japan increased the minimum age for vaccinations to two years. Following this, SIDS, spinal meningitis and other related nervous system diseases dramatically reduced and almost disappeared in Japan. Japan's ranking in infant mortality then went from being number 17 to being the country with the least infant mortalities in the world.

Research, which the AMA declined to support, suggests that SIDS is caused by excessive toxins and brain damage that the child receives due to vaccines.[32]

The patient information leaflet for the Wyeth DPT vaccine states that "The occurrence of SIDS has been reported following the administration of DPT" (but then, in typical drug-company-lawyer speak, the leaflet claims to not recognise the significance of the association of its vaccine with SIDS). But the leaflet does go on to helpfully point out that "The three primary doses of DPT are usually administered to infants between the ages of 2 and 6 months, and that approximately 85% of all SIDS cases occur in the periods 1 to 6 months, with peak incidence at ages 2-4 months."

Even though drug companies strive to distance the use of their vaccines from SIDS, the facts are clear. In chapters 5 and 6, it was shown the great lengths that drug companies go to to conceal the deaths caused by their drugs; it seems they also apply this same morality to their vaccines.

Data from the US Centers for Disease Control and Prevention confirms the above figures. In the US 10,000 babies die each year from SIDS. 85% of these deaths occur between the ages of 2-4 months. This age coincides with the initial DPT and polio inoculations.

Childhood cancer and leukaemia

Childhood cancer has been rising steadily in the US since the onset of mandatory vaccination programs in the 1950's. 62 Separate worldwide studies have linked the polio vaccine to brain tumours, bone cancers, lung lining cancers and leukaemia.[33]

Forbes Laurie, MD, of the Metro Cancer Hospital London, stated "I am convinced that the increase of cancer is due to vaccination."

Herbert Snow, MD, of the London Cancer Hospital, stated "I am convinced that some 80% of these cancer deaths are caused by smallpox vaccinations."

Other common adverse effects of vaccines

In 2002, the VAERS report to the US federal government included 244,424 reports of vaccine damage to children, which included the following: 99,145 emergency room visits; 5,149 life threatening reactions; 27,925 hospitalizations; 5,775 disabilities; and 5,309 deaths. When reading these figures, it should be remembered that the actual number of incidents would be very much higher, since the under-reporting of vaccine damage is acknowledged to be substantial. The FDA has stated that doctors under-report adverse vaccine reactions by 90%.[34] And a private Japanese study found that vaccine damage to children in England was 500 times under-reported.[35]

In 1994, a study published in the Journal of the American Medical Association showed that 11% of vaccinated children had asthma and developed pertussis (whooping cough), as compared to only 0.89% of unvaccinated children.

In 1997, a study published in the New Zealand Journal of Medicine, found that vaccinated populations of children had 23% more asthma and 30% more allergies compared to non-vaccinated children.

In 2000, the Feingold MD research group demonstrated that 26% of vaccinated children have asthma compared to only 2% of non-vaccinated children; and that 50% of vaccinated children had allergies compared to less than 1% of non-vaccinated children.

In 2002, a study in the Thorax Medical Journal showed that vaccinated children have 14 times more asthma and 10 times more eczema compared to non-vaccinated children.

In the so-called "gulf war syndrome", 275,000 British and US veterans became ill after the military campaign. In a later study, it was found that vaccinations were the main cause of their condition.[36]

The war on "germs", an alternative view

For almost 150 years, there has been a scientific debate on whether or not viruses and bacteria cause illness. Supported by hard evidence, a minority of scientists today believe that they do not, and that the central preoccupations of today's mainstream healthcare are misguided.

Working in 1878, Luis Pasteur is usually credited with coining the notion that "germs" may cause illness (though the notion existed for centuries before Pasteur's work). He also went on to produce failed vaccines for rabies and anthrax (p.129). In today's mainstream healthcare, Pasteur's ideas on "germ theory" still form the central notion of how diseases are caused.

However, working at the same time as Pasteur, was the scientist Pierre Bechamp. It is believed that Pasteur may have plagiarized most of Bechamp's work. Bechamp was known to be a quiet, humble man who shunned the limelight, which may explain why he was content for Pasteur to publically take credit for his work. But it was Bechamp who discovered the process of fermentation, which is usually cited as being one of Pasteur's greatest discoveries.

Bechamp studied live tissue (today's lab work is usually performed on dead tissue). In live tissue, he identified tiny bodies that he called Microzyma. He found these in both plant and animal tissue, and proposed that they were the basic units of life. In healthy tissue, they formed a normal part of the growing metabolism of cells. But in unhealthy, live tissue, he found that they evolved into bacteria. Hence, he discovered that bacteria are created within us. The type of microbe that the Microzyma evolved into depended on the surrounding environment within the tissue. This means that a particular bacteria or virus is created by our own tissue, to fulfil a particular need.

After the discovery of microzyma, Pierre Bechamps theorized that within the microscopic world, spontaneous generation occurs far more rapidly than in the gross, physical world. He witnessed these microzyma change shape at the earliest sign of an environmental shift. Microzyma are so pleomorphic (able to change shape) that Bechamp witnessed them change into virtually every viral, bacterial and fungal microbial shape known to science, simply by shifting the environment they existed in.[37]

This means that when our other immune cells, such as white blood cells and antibodies, cannot cope to clear particular toxins or other foreign bodies from our blood, these microzyma morph into the particular bacteria or virus that is needed to help destroy the toxin or foreign body. Therefore, when there is much toxicity in our blood, much bacteria will thus be created within us to help clear the toxic matter.

Alternatively, Pasteur claimed that bacteria have a fixed shape; are a single strain; and that they exist outside the body, and invade it to produce illness. This is the theory still adhered to today in mainstream healthcare. It relies on the pure supposition that just because micro-organisms are present when a person is ill, then those micro-organisms must have caused the illness. This is misguided, and also primitive thinking. At the time when (the plagiarist) Pasteur championed this notion, the evidence already existed to disprove it. Over a century ago, it was misguided supposition. Yet the notion has persisted.

Therefore when a doctor takes a culture from an ill patient, and finds bacteria present, he then prescribes antibiotics to try to kill the bacteria. This, of course, is the worst possible approach. The bacteria have been created within us to help clear toxic matter.

Bechamp's work suggests that any bacteria present, did not create your illness; nor did any virus, yeast, or any other natural microbe. These microbes arose from your own cells (today, they are called saprophytes) and are intended to help break down dead, diseased or dying organic matter.

During the time of bubonic plague, the approach used was the same as in today's mainstream healthcare. At the time, the living conditions were poor and congested, with no sanitation, lead piping supplied water, and the diet was poor. This created much toxicity within a person's blood, and they developed large, painful buboes glands (which gives the name to bubonic plague). The approach was to cut out what was "diseased," so the glands were removed from a person's arm pits and groin.

However, these glands are part of the lymphatic system, which is responsible for cleansing the blood, so it's not surprising that the glands went into overdrive. The patients lived in a highly toxic environment, and the physicians decided to cut out the glands that filtered their blood, so it's also not surprising that most such patients then died. Not much has changed in mainstream healthcare in 500 years.

Sanitation improved tremendously into the turn of the 20th century, which is why major infectious disease rates declined rapidly around 1910. And this was the only reason they declined. You could say disease rates declined despite mainstream healthcare, and certainly not because of it.

Bechamp's observations on live tissues were reproduced by many scientists through the early 1900's. And around the turn of the 20th century, an American scientist, Raymond Riffe, made technological advances that enabled greater insights. He developed a microscope using lenses made of quartz crystal, which allowed the full range of UV light to enter the scope; and he also greatly increased the magnification possible (to about 150,000 X). In live tissue, he found Bechamp's microzyma everywhere; and he found that these small units of life spontaneously evolved into varying forms of larger micro-organisms, depending on the type of tissue they existed in, healthy or toxic.[38]

Preceding this, in 1910, Dr H Rosenaeu showed that you can turn bacteria into different forms by altering their environment. He took a myriad of disease germs and placed them in the same media, and found that over time they all transformed into the same microorganism.[39]

In the 1953 textbook, Rational Bacteriology,[40] Bechamp's work was confirmed, and many experiments were cited that proved that micro-organisms like bacteria are formed from "granules" which are an inherent part of every living cell. When these granules transform into bacteria, they do so to boost immunity and aid the healing process. Staphylococci bacteria were found to be a primary force involved in the production of white blood cells for immunity against varying poisons, as well as generalized blood clotting. Hence, bacteria are produced within us, as a part of our body's defence, and are not fixed forms that invade us from outside to try to harm us. It has been shown that there are no fixed species of bacteria. A cocci can become a bacilli, a spirili, and vice versa; and they can also resolve into their smallest from, a sub-microscopic granule (which Bechamp called microzyma).

Whereas in today's mainstream healthcare, all such bacteria are imaged to be fixed forms, and to have invaded us from outside. Whenever they detect such bacteria in us, they attempt to wage war on these "germs" and wipe them out. This, of course, can only be harmful to the patient.

Today, Bechamps findings, which could be easily reproduced, are not investigated. When most funding and university research grants originate from drug companies, this is not surprising. No-one would expect a drug company to fund research that would undermine the very existence of the drug industry.

Chapter conclusion

The main point of the above is that the theory on "germs" is uncertain. Today, many doctors prescribe antibiotics as a cure-all, for just about any problem, even where the involvement of a bacterial infection could not possibly be the case. This is like an article of faith. Their medical thinking holds to this like a central tenet. The thinking goes something like, "Germs cause disease. Therefore if the person is unwell, this would most often be due to a germ, so prescribe an antibiotic." Very often, this might serve no purpose but to damage the health of the person, killing off the bacteria that are an essential element of their immune system.

The same is true of vaccination. The theory is uncertain. But in any case, it seems that artificially evoked antibodies provide no protection against the particular virus that they are intended to combat (p.130). Hence, immunized people will often contract the very disease the vaccine is supposed to protect them from, and on top of that, all people who receive the vaccine may suffer the potential adverse effects, which can sometimes be severe.

11. How do we become ill?

When a healthcare treatment is devised based on theorizing about how the body works, then that treatment is limited by the accuracy of the theory. As we saw in the chapters on the pharmaceutical approach and also on vaccines, this approach to healthcare has produced treatments that usually do not work and only harm the person's health.

The acupuncture developed by Chinese medicine over 2,000 years ago was discovered by making practical observations, and does not rely on any particular theory about how the body works (see page 33). And those practical observations encompass information about which organ malfunctions produce which symptoms, and what the mental and emotional causes of those organ malfunctions may be. This system, because it was not devised from any particular theory about how the body works, and has achieved over 2,000 years of consistent clinical results, provides the most reliable explanation for how we become ill.

The treatment itself utilizes the system of resonance between the main organs and body locations, which was formed throughout evolution.[1] This system of resonance, the "meridian system", is not a theoretical system. It is as real as the nervous or blood circulatory systems. And during the treatment, nothing foreign to the body is introduced, and no mechanism in the body is hampered, on any level (unlike today's approach, which chemically blocks healthy functions in a misguided attempt to improve health). Also, no direct attempt is made to manipulate systems in the body (based on theories about those systems); the "meridian system" is stimulated simply to prompt the related organ to itself make whatever adjustments are necessary on the chemical level (for example), to return the organ to normal function. Hence, the system of acupuncture does not itself encompass, or rely on, any ideas about how we become ill. Those ideas are embodied in the ancient practical observations.

Why Use Natural Healing?

Inappropriate thoughts cause illness

In ancient China, it was observed that many of the more serious symptoms people suffer are caused by inappropriate thought patterns. These disrupt the function of the main organs, and it is these malfunctions in the main organs that produce the symptoms. The main such symptoms related to each organ are listed on pages 9 to 13.

There are some apparent exceptions to this rule. For example, a child may be born with organ malfunctions, inherited from their parents (as frequently happens with poor kidney function). In this case, the initial cause would lie with the inappropriate thought patterns of the child's parents; but once a child has such organ malfunctions themselves, this tends to produce the same inappropriate thought patterns in them, so that the same rule applies; it is those inappropriate thought patterns that cause or (in this case) perpetuate the organ malfunction, and this malfunction then produces all the symptoms that the person suffers.

In developed countries, the organ most commonly affected is probably the liver. This is because the types of stress that are common in the workplace and in life in general tend to cause us to adopt thought patterns that stagnate our liver function. When this continues for any time and becomes pronounced, this could produce any of the symptoms listed on page 10.

Many of these symptoms are powerful, such as constant anger, cramps, stiff neck and shoulders, depression, paranoia, migraines or headaches, period cramps, PMS. This is because the liver is a powerful organ and it has a big influence on many aspects of our body. The key to properly healing any of these symptoms (and also the other, less powerful liver-related symptoms), is to return the liver to normal function. As with all the organs, this is achieved in seconds with acupuncture. When the liver function is stagnated, key liver-related acupoints would feel very tender when pressed. This is because those locations are reflecting the stress that is currently in the person's liver. By stimulating any of these points with acupuncture, this encourages the tissue at that point to return to normal, and in turn (due to the resonance between the liver and this location), this then encourages the liver to also release its stress and return to normal function. This happens within seconds during the treatment, which I have verified countless times by using all the diagnostic techniques available to a traditional acupuncturist. This explains why the patient usually feels so deeply relaxed at the end of the treatment; they feel this way because their main organs have released the stress that they were used to living with.

As with all the organs, when the liver function is returned to normal, this would remove the tendency to adopt the type of thought patterns that stagnate the liver function, so that the person's previous symptoms would not tend to return. But with the liver in particular, the associated thought patterns can be addictive, or difficult to escape, so when the person returns to their life and all the same situations, some people immediately return to adopting the same damaging thought patterns, which then stagnates their liver function again, and the previous symptoms return. This would usually only happen with people who are unusually stubborn. They cannot escape the self destructive pattern they were used to.

The most common inappropriate liver-related thought pattern is the tendency to be too controlling. The person has the desire to control every aspect of their life, including their own behaviour and that of all the people around them. This controlling is what the liver does within our own body, controlling and organizing the creation of our energy and the movement of resources around our body. When this liver function is used by our conscious mind, this is what produces all our thoughts about how other people should behave. And what causes the problem for the person's own liver function is when other people, objects, or society decline to obey the person's ideas about how they should behave. It is this "refusal to conform to the person's wishes" that blocks the person's liver-related thoughts, and hence immediately blocks the function of their own liver. When their liver function is blocked (or stagnated), the liver then produces any of the powerful symptoms mentioned before.

The approach of today's mainstream healthcare to any of these symptoms, would be to see each individual symptom as the problem, and attempt to chemically block the healthy function of a system in the

Why Use Natural Healing?

body (not related to the liver) to attempt to prevent the symptom from appearing; but without tackling the real, underlying problem, and usually not even being aware of what the real problem is. This is not healthcare, is certainly not healing, and only worsens the health of the person, not only by not addressing the real issue, but by chemically blocking an unrelated, and healthy part of the person's body, which could then only create further health problems for the person in future—on top of the original condition, which is left untreated.

The same situation is true of the other main organs, the pancreas, lungs, heart, and kidneys. Each of these organ functions is capable of being used by our conscious mind to process our thoughts. The type of thoughts related to each organ, mimic the organ's physical function in our body; and this explains the close relationship between those organ functions and the related thought patterns (pp.17-24). And with each, it is possible to overuse a particular thought pattern, which then disrupts the physical function of the related organ, and it is this disruption (or poor function), that then causes the organ to produce the symptoms we suffer.

This process explains how all the symptoms listed on pages 9 to 13 usually result. And returning the related organ to normal function with acupuncture hence clears any of those symptoms.

In clinic, patients often respond with amazement when a long-standing health problem is suddenly cleared with acupuncture. I have seen this often with conditions like hay fever and asthma, where the person's life has been heavily affected by the condition, but then the condition is suddenly not there. As a healer, this outcome seems normal. The healing is achieved by simply treating the appropriate organ. But when the patient has spent years using the drug remedy approach (which only chemically blocks the function of a healthy system in their body not related to the underlying cause, such as with antihistamines or inhalers*), the sudden healing of their condition can seem miraculous.

---

*These block the normal function of the smooth muscle of the airways in the lungs. See page 135.

Infectious conditions

The ancient Chinese physicians recognised that we could be affected by external, physical pathogens. These pathogens could include cold, dampness or "wind". These ideas do not correspond exactly with pathogens in today's terminology.[2] But the important concept is that Chinese medicine recognises that we can be affected by our environment; and this idea would equate to today's notion of infectious diseases, such as the common cold or flu, or similar conditions.

An important concept in Chinese medicine is that not all people who are exposed to the same external pathogen get ill. It is only the people whose resilience is lower, who would become ill. But with a strong and healthy person, they would not be affected in the same way by the same pathogen.

Their approach to treating a common cold or flu would be to use acupoints that treat a particular aspect of the lungs, and also its more "superficial", related organ, the large intestine. There were ancient theories to attempt to explain how such a treatment works, but these tended to be metaphorical ideas; and the important thing is that the treatment returns aspects of our main organs back to normal, and our normal defences are then able to protect us from the pathogen. If the treatment is applied early enough, this is usually enough to prevent the cold or flu from developing at all.

Hence, as to whether or not you are affected by seasonal flu, or similar conditions, it all depends on how well you are. If you are stressed, run down, or have a weak constitution, your normal defences would probably be unable to protect you, and you become ill.

A marked example of just such a pathogen was the 2020 respiratory pandemic. When a person contracted this virus and struggled to overcome it, the natural healing approach would be to treat the person's lungs, returning them to normal function; and also treating their "kidney" function. In Chinese medicine, it is recognised that the "kidney" function needs to be good to enable our lungs to breathe in; and the "kidneys" (which include the adrenal glands) is also the key organ that supports our immunity. Provided the patient was not taking drugs that chemically blocked aspects of the organs from working normally, then there is no reason why all such patients who were treated with natural healing should not be able to fight off the pathogen and quickly return to good health.

However, in all developed countries, today's mainstream healthcare is unable to return an organ to normal function (simply because it has no knowledge of how to do this). Hence it could not treat such a simple condition, and the whole world was brought to its knees due to this ineptitude; and in the meantime, mainstream healthcare became obsessed with doing battle with a virus, which was the only option it had left itself since it was not capable of doing normal healing. But as demonstrated in Chapter 10, the panic to develop a vaccine was a red herring.

Redness, rashes and skin eruptions

In Chinese medicine, such conditions are recognised as simply being an expression of a stressed state in the organ whose meridian the anomaly appears on. Hence, rather than considering this to be due to a bacterial "infection", or similar, the superficial condition is not treated directly, but instead the related organ is treated to return it to normal function, and then the redness, rash, or eruption clears, since the organ is now functioning normally.

A good demonstration of this principle is the signs that appear on a person's tongue to reflect the health of their organs. The states in all the organs are continuously reflected to particular aspects of the tongue. When the organs are functioning normally, there are no anomalies on the tongue. But when an organ is stressed, the area of the tongue related to that organ may appear reddened. This redness is not due to an infection, or injury of any kind on the tongue; it is simply reflecting the state in the related organ.

This is confirmed in clinic. Common examples that I have noticed are redness in the heart or liver regions on the tongue. When I have seen this, and then treated the related organ with acupuncture, then re-checked the tongue, the redness usually clears completely (or sometimes greatly diminishes) within seconds of the needle being inserted in an acupoint related to that organ. This is an experimental confirmation that the redness on the tongue was reflecting the real-time state in the related organ function.

The same is true of anomalies that appear on the body, in the region of a particular meridian. This might include redness, swelling; or the skin feeling warm or cold to the touch. These are not due to bacterial or viral "infections". And this is also confirmed during a treatment. When the related organ is treated with acupuncture, to return its function to normal, these anomalies on its meridian usually clear within seconds. Such anomalies are not due to an injury or local "infection" of any sort. Instead, they can be viewed as providing a valuable diagnostic indicator of which organ is stressed.

Another common example of this principle is a sore throat. In Chinese medicine, it is recognised that a sore throat is simply a reflection of a particular state in the lungs. This might be an injury to the lungs due to breathing in an external pathogen. This does not mean that this pathogen is directly producing the sore throat. But rather, the lungs are stressed in a certain way, and this state is reflected to the tissue at the throat, resulting in a sore throat. There are no "germs" involved at the throat, at least no "invading germs". The proof of this is in the routine acupuncture treatment. Acupoints are used to treat this aspect of lung "stress", mainly Lung-5, or Lung-10. Both these acupoints would be tender when pressed, which reflects the state in the lungs that is producing the sore throat. When either of these acupoints is needled, the lungs return to normal function and the patient's sore throat clears within seconds. This would include any reddened or swollen tissue in the area of the sore throat. The fact that these anomalies clear within seconds, confirms that "invading germs" are not the cause of the sore throat.

According to the Bechamp school of thought (p.140), as a part of the body's immunity, bacteria would usually be created from within us when the tissue at any location experiences an anomalous state. This is a normal and essential part of the body's own immunity. The theory is that these bacteria are created to help clear any damaged or dead cells. Our own white blood cells normally perform this function, but they require the assistance of these extra micro-organisms to perform the task.

Mainstream healthcare, which only thinks in terms of "invading germs", would take a swab of the throat, find bacteria there, and leap to the wrong conclusion that the whole illness (sore throat) is the result of "invading bacteria", and prescribe antibiotics, which then only interferes with the body's normal healing and maintenance processes; and does nothing to return the lungs to normal function (in other words, does not help the lungs to heal properly).

As regards the microbiology of the body, the whole story is not fully understood; and appears to be mainly misunderstood by mainstream healthcare. When micro-organisms where discovered in the body, such as bacteria, fungi, viruses, in line with the prevailing "germ theory" of Luis Pasteur, they were mistakenly thought to be alien to the body, rather than an integral part of it. And this mistaken notion has informed the thinking of mainstream healthcare ever since. But natural healing is far more effective, and does no damage to the patient, because it is far closer to understanding how the body works—ironically, because it "stands back" and takes a wider view.

The fact that natural healing does not need to understand the part played by microorganisms (such as bacteria, fungi, viruses), turns out to be an advantage. It is not trying to meddle with this part of the person, therefore it does not need to understand it anyway. It uses the same mechanism in the body that produces most symptoms (and is thought to have even caused the evolution of the body[3]). It "nudges" this mechanism, to cause the body to heal itself, and do this rapidly, and without causing any harm to the person. A treatment having "adverse effects" is a concept peculiar to drug remedies, and was created by drug companies to attempt to make "adverse effects" seem like a normal part of "medicine".

Painful joints, tendons and muscles

The same mechanism mentioned above, which causes the states of our organs to be reflected in the tissue along each organ's related meridian, also frequently causes such things as painful or stiff joints, tendons or muscles. The central concept involved is called the intelligent tissue theory, which states that all bodily tissue is able to interpret organ information conveyed on electromagnetic waves.[4] This mechanism explains how the organ stress is communicated to the distal tissue at any location on the related organ's meridian. The mechanism was only described and demonstrated in 2018-19, which is perhaps one of the reasons why today's mainstream healthcare is unaware of the mechanism.

A common such joint pain is at the hip. The gallbladder meridian runs through the hip. The gallbladder is functionally very closely related to the liver, and prolonged stagnated liver function, induced by many types of stress, can often manifest as stiffness and pain of the hip. This clears immediately when the liver function is corrected with acupuncture. I have frequently found that patients who have experienced stiff hips for some time, when they stand from my treatment couch, and their stiffness and pain is no longer there, they find it miraculous and almost start skipping and jumping. The caveat is that if they are taking drug remedies, the treatment will not last, since the organs cannot maintain their normal function while the body's chemistry is being blocked with drugs. Also, the person needs to accept the mental adjustments that the treatment will be encouraging them to make. This often means trying to be much less controlling than is their habit. If they slip right back into the same, damaging mental habits, the liver function will again quickly become permanently stagnated, and all the related symptoms will reappear.

In mainstream healthcare, they are unaware of all these mechanisms (despite the fact that the mechanisms have been well known for over 2,000 years, and have been seen in clinic with consistent results over all that time), and instead they rely on high tech devices to look at the tissue around the joint. As soon as they see any anomaly, they wrongly conclude that that anomaly is the problem, which usually means they would recommend surgery to replace the joint. The patient might even be shown a scan, with the technician pointing to the anomaly, and be told something like, "Your hip joint is worn out; it needs to be replaced." Yet, in many of these instances, surgery is totally unnecessary; and a much more medically-advanced solution (ironically) would be to use ancient, natural healing. In comparison, it would not be unfair to regard the approach of today's mainstream healthcare as misguided and primitive.

With many such anomalies, these are more likely to be the result of this same mechanism, and simply reflecting the stressed state in the related organ, so that the anomaly may also heal once the organ function had been corrected. But mainstream healthcare sees the anomaly and wrongly assumes that this is the problem.

I have also often seen this same situation in regard to certain wrist pains, primarily around the thumb joint. In the instances I've seen, the wrist pain is a reflection of damage to the lungs, caused by a previous bereavement, usually about a year previous to the wrist pain starting. In Chinese medicine it is recognised that the lung function is damaged when the person experiences a bereavement. Once the person is recovering from their bereavement, and their lungs begin to recover from this damage, the "pain" is released from the lungs, moving towards the outside of the lungs. The lung meridian is located along the arm, and the progress of this pain as it exits the lungs is reflected to a location along the lung meridian, more and more towards the tip of the meridian (at the thumb), as it progresses towards the surface of the lungs. This pain often gets "stuck" at a strong lung acupoint, Lung-9, at the base of the thumb. And this is the cause of the pain and stiffness. It could remain at this location for only a few days, or weeks or months, depending on the person. The natural healing solution is to further treat the lungs with acupuncture, to help heal the remaining damage caused by the person's bereavement. In mainstream healthcare, the solution may be to perform surgery on the wrist; again, unnecessarily.

This same mechanism (the intelligent tissue theory), can account for many such joint, tendon or muscle pains. The solution is usually to locate the meridian where the pain is situated, treat the related organ with acupuncture, and the symptoms then usually clear within that same treatment session. Often acupoints are used on that same meridian, near to where the pain is located, but this also amounts to treating the related organ.

This same mechanism can account for many types of injury. I have even experienced healing a hernia with acupuncture, and the healing was confirmed with an ultrasound scan.[5] In this instance, the treatment enabled the patient to avoid surgery.

Lifestyle factors

Our body is designed to work properly under "normal" conditions. This means when getting a reasonable amount of exercise each day, and eating or drinking appropriate foods. If this is not done, then our main organs cannot function at their best, and this will produce symptoms.

In particular, the liver is heavily affected by insufficient physical activity. Often this inactivity is also accompanied by stress (such as sitting all day at work under the stress of the job), and this type of stress also causes the liver function to further stagnate, adding to the possible symptoms.

Eating too much, and often too much of the wrong types of food, is another cause of ill health. The pancreas is the other most commonly affected organ in the developed world. The pancreas function is weakened by too much thinking. Its function peaks at eleven a.m., which is when we would ideally eat our largest meal of the day. After this time, we should only eat smaller amounts, occasionally. But today, society is usually organized so that we eat our largest meal in the evening, when our digestion is at its weakest. And we do this after thinking all day long in relation to our work or studies, so that our pancreas and stomach functions are already weakened, when we then overload our digestion even further with a full meal. This pattern is a recipe for ill health. When we are young, our digestion is much stronger and we can cope with this lifestyle, but by our late twenties or thirties, it cannot be sustained while remaining healthy.

The wrong types of foods are also often advocated by today's mainstream healthcare. It suggests that raw vegetables are more healthy, but this is nonsense. It observes that an uncooked carrot has more vitamins than a cooked one. But if your pancreas function is too weak to digest raw vegetables, you obtain no nutrition from the food, and eating raw vegetables only weakens your pancreas further, increasing such symptoms as IBS. Another bad habit is drinking chilled water or other liquids. When we swallow a chilled liquid, this shocks our stomach, and hence weakens its function. If you are a sensitive person, when you drink a chilled liquid, you will be aware of a cold shock shooting down the stomach meridian on your abdomen (at about five cm on either side of your belly button). This is a reflection of the pain felt by your stomach organ.

Food and liquids should be cooked and warm. And heavy thinking or worrying should be reserved for the early morning, when your digestion is at its peak; and avoided for the remainder of the day. If this is not done, you will be weakening your stomach and pancreas function, producing such symptoms as IBS (p.9), and you will be unable to extract adequate nutrition from the food you do eat, which will also be detrimental to your health.

Another bad habit promoted by mainstream healthcare is the avoidance of salt. Salt is an essential nutrient, required for good "kidney" function; it also improves the flavour and enjoyment of food, which enjoyment itself enhances our health.

When observing today's mainstream healthcare, and their related ideas on food, I am reminded that too little knowledge is certainly a dangerous thing. Today's "food science" may also claim that food cooked or warmed in a microwave oven is just as "healthy" as food cooked in a conventional oven. Such statements only reveal the inadequacy of their knowledge. When food is microwaved, this destroys the flavour of the food, which indicates that it has destroyed a vital element of the food's nutrition (even though "food scientists" may be unable to measure this). The result of this type of misinformation is that large numbers of people are eating microwaved food with hardly any seasoning, at the time of day when their digestion is at its weakest, and after a day of stress and inactivity. All these factors are detrimental to their health. And if they were to consult a doctor, a few pharmaceuticals may be added, chemically blocking the function of their main organs. Hence, today's mainstream healthcare (together with its "food science") is another major cause of illness.

12. Why has an inept, misguided system been adopted by mainstream healthcare?

The previous chapters show the mainstream drug-based approach to healthcare to be a system that is ineffective and responsible for greatly harming the health of millions of people every year. It is primitive, unscientific, and sustained by widespread fraud on the part of drug companies, and also propaganda which wrongly convinces the media, politicians, many scientists, and the majority of the world population that their practice is advanced, modern, scientific, evidence based, safe and effective, in the manner of a glorious but fake medical religion. The ideas are clearly appealing. But why is the message so appealing, and why is it believed? In short, how on earth has such a damaging system persisted for so long, and become so all-powerful?

To understand why the thinking behind mainstream healthcare is (in effect) propaganda, and to understand why that propaganda is so convincing to doctors, patients and the media, it is necessary to look at how the system evolved, and to identify the fallacies at each stage, and clear up the misunderstandings that have since become accepted truths.

How did it all start?

There is a long history of different medial ideas and approaches, stretching from ancient China, Egypt and India, to today. It is most instructive to put aside theories on how the body works (which are often untrue or incomplete, whichever period they originate from, including today), and consider the purely practical aspect of medicine.

For over 2,000 years, medical practices consisted mainly of prescribing herbs or spices, which, through experiment, were discovered to have healing effects. Traditional acupuncture, which is my own area of expertise, achieved healing by stimulating locations on the body which were found to be related to the main organs and could return those organs to normal function merely by stimulating these related locations. This same mechanism is able to explain why some types of massage can also achieve similar healing. This knowledge, and the ability to make accurate diagnoses of which organ is involved in the production of certain symptoms, was developed and refined over thousands of years, and remains remarkably accurate today.

These healing modalities were all based on practical observations, rather than on theorizing about how the body works, then using those theories to make adjustments to the body to attempt to improve the patient's health. And these healthcare systems worked perfectly over all that time, as long as theorizing did not get in the way.

Over the past few hundred years, as large cities formed, many people lived in squalid conditions and this naturally caused much disease, for whatever reason. And once living conditions were improved, the health and life expectancy of people also dramatically improved. Again, there is no certainty about the reasons for this. Rather than the main reason being related to any particular version of germ theory, I believe it is more likely to be related to the mental health of the people. When people are happy and have relatively little stress, they will be much more healthy. In my own acupuncture practice, I have always noted that most diseases (including most chronic illnesses) have their origin in mental and emotional aspects of the person (leaving aside the conditions inadvertently caused by today's prescribed drugs). Of course there are toxic substances in the environment that can damage us. These too were reduced in societies over the last century or so, and this would have played its own part in improving health.

The seeds of today's mainstream medical approach were sowed during this last century. After the discovery of the microscope and advances in chemistry, this led to a shift in the mainstream approach to healthcare. Now, theorizing about how the body works and becomes ill, is the new guiding principle. And most treatments are designed according to these theories.

12. Why has an inept, misguided system been adopted by mainstream healthcare?

Today's approach needed dishonestly to validate it

The practice of vaccination perhaps marked a turning point in the evolution of today's mainstream healthcare approach. It proved controversial from the start, and perhaps set the tone regarding the conduct of drug companies, most doctors, and the creation of medical propaganda.

From the beginning, it was clear that the theory was not borne out by the results. The vaccinations only increased the instance of the target disease, by causing the disease in many people (p.124), and often produced severe adverse effects. But by this time, the drug industry was already big business, so corporate publicists produced propaganda to support drug company profits (which, of course, is only to be expected from big corporate organizations). Where possible, the harmful effects of their vaccines were concealed (p.136), scaremongering was devised about the dreadful, crippling "germs" (such as polio) and lies were told about how the miracle of vaccination had "eradicated" these dreadful diseases; whereas many of the infectious diseases of the previous century (including polio) had declined naturally, before mass vaccination programs began (p.124); and vaccination had only increased the incidence of the target diseases (pp.125, 127, and 128).

Through the history of vaccination, despite the evidence of the harm done and the false claims of drug companies (claiming credit for "eradicating" diseases that had cleared prior to their vaccines being used, and only increased afterwards), the theory of vaccination was taught to all medical students, and it seemed to make sense, so doctors repeated it. Drug companies lied about the effectiveness and covered up the harms, and doctors (whose main source of information is drug companies) believed the lies; what else could they do? And even health authorities bent the facts to support the accepted theory of vaccination (p.124). After all, health authorities were manned by (or advised by) doctors, who were trained in the theory of vaccination, which made sense to them, and was derived from the theory of how the immune system works, so that a large part of their medical thinking supported the theory of vaccination. To doctors, this all made sense, because it was a central part of their professional belief system. And because this made sense to them, they would naturally conclude that it must be true. Therefore the health authorities needed to bend the facts to make them support the theory. What else, they might say, could they do? Were the medical textbooks untrue; were the doctors all lying; were the drug companies lying? If so, the only explanation may be that the drug companies were perpetrating a massive fraud, which was being covered up by doctors. The health authorities, understandably, were perhaps not brave enough to face that possibility, so they supported the drug companies and doctors, and produced fake "evidence" and further propaganda concerning the efficacy and safety of vaccines (p.124).

Hence, the party line became "vaccination is safe and effective", which is towed today, by doctors, drug companies, politicians, and the media. And the message was believed by most people. After all, this is the age of science, so it must be correct. But what people did not realize is that this was not science. The scientific method had long-since been abandoned by the medical industry. This is most vividly seen in relation to drug remedies.

The complete abandonment of scientific principles

In 1957, the first modern, notable drug disaster began, with thalidomide (p.62). The drug was promoted for morning sickness, though the company knew of the birth defects it caused. For sixteen years, the drug company fought to conceal the devastating harms of the drug, while continuing to promote it as a safe drug.

After this disaster, the regulatory authorities began demanding that drug companies trialled their drugs before they would be licensed. From here, the conduct of drug companies only declined.

As seen in chapters 5 to 7, it became routine for drug companies to report fake trial results. Either a drug trial was designed with bias built in, to produce the required outcome; or the data was manipulated to produce a fake positive result for the trial drug, to replace the negative result that their trial had produced.

12. Why has an inept, misguided system been adopted by mainstream healthcare?

This conduct was adopted as the norm, because when a trial was conducted and analysed scientifically, it usually demonstrated that the trial drug did not work, therefore science had to be abandoned, in favour of massive profits and at the expense of consumer healthcare.

Along with this fraud, a propaganda smoke screen was created to make the industry seem scientific and to wrongly convince doctors, the media and the public that drugs were effective and that this was "evidence based medicine," which it certainly was not.

Statistics also started to be used to help to further conceal the truth. In statistics, there is something called a "P" value. This simply means the probability that the results of a trial did not happen by chance. It has become accepted that a P value of 0.04 or less can be taken as proof that the results were real. This simply means that, statistically, there is a 96% chance that the results did not happen by chance. In this case, the results are said to be "statistically significant". This comment is often made of a drug trial outcome. To most doctors and laymen, this comment would be interpreted to mean that the drug produces significant results. However, it means nothing of the sort. It is making no comment on the performance of the drug, only on the structure of the trial. And as shown on page 81, only a very small amount of dishonest data manipulation is required to obtain such a P number in most trials, however "insignificant" the results might actually have been.

The fact that most doctors (and certainly most lay people) do not understand drugs, drug trials, or statistics, is used to the advantage of drug companies. Claims can be made that seem impressive to the lay person, but which are not really saying anything at all. People are "blinded by statistics".

But even when the data is analysed honestly, the positive outcome for the trail drug is often only around 10%, or even much less when such factors as bias are taken into account (p.82). What this means is that if 100 people took the drug, less than 10 of them would notice an improvement in their condition, however slight; and in the other 90 people, there would be no improvement, and they would still have to suffer all the adverse effects of the drug. Yet the results of such a trial would still obtain a P value indicating the results were "statistically significant".

When looked at in reality, like this, no-one in their right mind would consider it acceptable to prescribe such a drug. But it is even worse in reality. Such trials are in the minority. It is more common for such a meagre outcome to be fictional. As demonstrated in Chapter 6, only a tiny amount of fraud is required to turn a negative result into a positive one, in favour of the trial drug; and when the legitimate results of a trial prove that the drug does not work, it has been shown that drug companies are prepared to fake the results, for purely commercial reasons (pp.63-67). With such a drug, this means that near to 100% of the people who take it will only suffer the adverse effects, and experience no improvement in their condition.

It is so easy to manipulate trial data in this way to produce fake outcomes that "prove" a drug works, that this has given rise to the drug company practice of taking a drug that was designed for one condition, and applying it to many other conditions (which its method of action could not conceivably have an effect on), and producing a fake trial result wrongly claiming to "prove" it works for these other conditions (p.84). The motivation is purely commercial, to sell as many drugs as possible, to as many people as possible, even though the drugs have no benefit for them and only harm them.

In such a climate, the drug companies claim that this is "evidence based medicine", and is "scientific". When you have to fake the evidence, you cannot legitimately claim that the practice is "evidence based". Such descriptions as "evidence based medicine" and "scientific" and "drugs are tested and proved to be safe and effective", these are all pure propaganda, but are repeated by doctors and the media, who simply trust that the drug industry is honest.

In this climate, another propaganda device of drug companies was to invent the notion of the "placebo effect". It was common for a drug to be shown to have an effect in only a very small percentage of patients (assuming the trial results were legitimate). Therefore, this placebo effect was invented, which claimed that giving someone a neutral, inac-

12. Why has an inept, misguided system been adopted by mainstream healthcare?

tive pill would improve their condition in around 50% of people, so that by prescribing the active drug, which only worked in perhaps 5% of people, around 55% of people may be claimed to gain some benefit from it, due to this invented placebo effect.

This is propaganda, created to cast a smoke screen over the fact that most drugs produce very little, if any, positive effect in most people; and to justify the prescribing of such drugs. In reality, that 50% improvement that is often seen in drug trials among the group who did not take the active drug, simply happened when people were not treated at all, due to the condition spontaneously improving, which only confirmed that it was better to not prescribe any drugs at all (p.108). However, doctors and the media accept at face value what the drug companies tell them. Now, the "placebo effect" is accepted to be a real phenomenon, even though it has been shown that it does not exist, to any real extent (p.79). It is pure myth.

This myth does form part of the armoury of mainstream healthcare in another way. When doctors hear of any natural healing that produces good results, particularly in areas where mainstream healthcare is incapable of achieving anything similar, their usual response is to dismiss the real healing as "placebo". All their training is unable to understand this healing, so they dismiss it as having no effect, and wrongly imagine that the healing was done by the person's own mind, simply because the person believed they would get better.

Hence, this invented placebo concept provides medics with a way of dismissing anything beyond their knowledge. And all the above dishonest techniques used by drug companies serve to wrongly convince doctors that mainstream healthcare is "evidence based" and that most drugs are "safe and effective." But there is an even more important factor that tends to produce a delusional mindset in doctors.

How do doctors become convinced that their approach to healthcare is normal?

When a doctor does not have the knowledge that a healer has, and the doctor's conduct to their patients is only damaging to the patient's health when considered in the light of the healer's knowledge, it can be difficult to understand the doctor's point of view. Therefore, to be able to understand today's healthcare, and why doctors think it is normal to do what they do, you need to put out of your mind all knowledge of real healing, and then consider the approach of doctors.

What knowledge does natural healing have that is absent from today's mainstream medical knowledge? The Chinese medicine knowledge of how subtle malfunctions in our main organs produce most of the symptoms that people routinely suffer, and why those organs malfunction, this knowledge was discovered over 2,000 years ago and has remained consistent and accurate to this day. The symptoms related to each organ were described on pages 9 to 13. Many of these associations are still unknown in today's physiology.

For example, this Chinese-medicine branch of natural healing is aware that most cases of asthma are due to poor function of the "kidneys"; that the symptoms of IBS are caused by poor pancreas function; that the symptoms of a migraine are produced by stagnated liver function; that a good sense of smell and a strong voice, requires good lung function; that many aspects of eyesight are dependent on good liver function; and that many of the other associations between common symptoms and a particular organ (pp.9-13) are directly produced by poor function of that organ. Yet there is no knowledge in today's physiology that can account for most of these mechanisms. The organ functions are simply not understood in enough detail to be able to account for all the symptoms produced when the organ has a subtle malfunction, and there is also little understanding of most of those malfunctioning states. In other words, most of the subtle malfunctions that are routinely detected and treated in traditional acupuncture could not even be detected with today's diagnostic tests or examinations. And importantly, when considering the routine interaction between our main organs and our thoughts, which causes many of these subtle malfunctions in our main organs (pp.16-24), there is not even a branch of today's physiology that is aware of this mechanism, let alone having studied or understood it.

12. Why has an inept, misguided system been adopted by mainstream healthcare?

All this medical knowledge was discovered merely by making practical observations in ancient China, but it has recently been shown that acupuncture can be explained by the intelligent tissue theory (p.153). This involves organ information being conveyed on electromagnetic waves, to every location in our body and beyond (which also explains how we can be aware of when nearby people are stressed; and it even enables us to feel certain of their symptoms which are duplicated in us). In order for today's physiology to understand all these associations between subtle organ malfunctions and symptoms known in Chinese medicine, it is possible that it may need to understand this communication method, which it so far has no knowledge of at all. Organ information conveyed in this way can account for many subtle phenomena that cannot be explained using today's physiology.

Apart from this knowledge of the underlying cause of most symptoms, today's mainstream healthcare also has no knowledge of how to correct these subtle organ malfunctions that occur routinely as part of living in the modern world. Mostly, they are even unaware when a particular organ is malfunctioning anyway (since this type of malfunction is too subtle to show up in today's diagnostic tests). Whereas, with traditional acupuncture, it is clear which organ malfunction is producing all the patient's symptoms; and that organ can be easily and immediately returned to normal function, which then clears all the symptoms, and also makes the person feel great, because their main organs are no longer stressed.

If you take away all the above knowledge, what is left?

When a patient complains of a symptom, the real underlying cause (which organ is functioning poorly to produce that symptom, and why the organ adopted this malfunction) is unknown to the doctor. Instead they are only able to see the symptom in isolation, as a separate problem in itself.

Today's physiology has managed to identify the basics of how chemicals are used for communication in the body. And it so happens that many of these communication mechanisms can be blocked by designing a specific chemical to prevent the communication from happening (pp.33-37). Since these blocking chemicals can be easily mass produced, this technique lends itself readily to today's drug industry. In many health situations, there is the opportunity to chemically block a normal healthy function of some aspect of the body which then prevents a particular symptom from appearing. This is the case with blood-pressure related issues (p.37), with asthma (p.116), period-related issues, hay fever (p.182), migraine, some joint and muscle pains, and many other symptoms.

If you were only to see the symptom as the problem, then the above approach would seem to have solved the problem. But in reality, this approach amounts to a chemical trick being played on the body to temporarily conceal the symptom; and this trick has chemically blocked a normal, healthy function in the body, and also accidentally produced a blocking effect on most of the main organ functions (p.58), all of which can only impede the patient's health in the long term.

But today's healthcare would not be aware of this issue. As explained above, today's mainstream healthcare tends to only see the symptom and not the underlying cause, because with most common symptoms (pp.9-13), there is nothing in its knowledge to identify an organ malfunction that could produce that particular symptom. Doctors can only be aware of what their training tells them. Therefore, in their minds, the reality is that the symptom *is* the problem.

Another way to put this is as follows. Because today's physiology has focused on studying the body at the microscopic level, this has tended to dictate that the mainstream approach to healthcare has become to attempt to make changes to the body on the microscopic level to attempt to correct health issues. But due to the limited knowledge, this usually only results in them damaging the person's health.

Why is it regarded as normal to harm patients?

It is this accidental and (in effect) random blocking of organ functions that probably produces all the known adverse effects of drugs, and also the unknown effects (such as the future complications). But by the introduction of the notion of "side effects", the drug industry has created the notion that it is normal for drugs to produce harm. In other words

12. Why has an inept, misguided system been adopted by mainstream healthcare?

(from the doctor's point of view), it is normal for "medicine" to harm the patient.

This probably explains why this notion of "side effects" is, in doctors' minds, also wrongly extended to herbal treatments. On page 31, I described a misconception that most people have about the nature of drugs. They tend to regard them as generally being similar in nature to herbal remedies; that both herbs and drugs are simply pills or potions taken in response to illness, and work in similar ways. This could not be more wrong. But this misconception probably also exists in the minds of most doctors. And because doctors have accepted that medicine could harm the patient, they also assume that herbs can also produce such "side effects". In the usual sense, this is impossible, because herbs do not chemically block healthy function. They do not chemically block any function. This blocking action is a "trick" performed by today's drug industry, which is why adverse effects are peculiar to drugs.

Another way to look at this, is that this is the only approach drug companies can use, due to the limitation of drug design. In medical school, doctors are indoctrinated in this approach. They are taught the mechanisms used by common drugs. With almost all common drugs, this approach consists of chemically blocking a normal and healthy aspect of the body, to attempt to conceal a symptom (pp.31-58). The teaching of this approach makes it seem to the medical student like a normal thing to do. And as doctors, they hence think this is normal, is healthcare, is "medicine". Once such blocking drugs are designed, they are then applied at random to treat other conditions, just to see if this blocking of particular chemistry just happens to produce an effect in another area of the body that can be considered a benefit (p.84). This approach is also accepted as normal by the medical student. And because mainstream healthcare has now got to the stage where healthcare *is* the drug industry, then no other options are considered to be available. The job of being a doctor then becomes a balance between attempting to produce a "benefit," and the harm done to the patient.

In reality, that "benefit" is often fictitious, and a product of drug company misinformation. But doctors usually take at face value what drug companies tell them, and what health authorities tell them. And when this information is misleading, you could say that most doctors are tricked into routinely harming patients. When they tow the party line, and indulge in the thinking introduced by drug companies, they recite such concepts as "the benefit outweighs the harm," and a drug being "well tolerated," and "drugs are tested and found to be safe and effective," in this "evidence based medicine." Yet, these concepts are all untrue and pure propaganda.

Statistical smoke screens
Another statistical concept that is used to convince doctors that this drug approach to healthcare is normal, is that of "number needed to treat" or NNT. This describes the number of patients that must be treated before one of them will gain some benefit from the drug. In real healthcare, such a number would always be "one." In other words, every patient treated would benefit from the treatment. But in drug-company-sponsored healthcare a NNT of five or ten would be common; and with some drugs, the number is around fifty or higher. This, for example, might mean that if a drug is given to fifty people for (say) five years, then (statistically) one of those people might be prevented from having a heart attack; and it is acceptable that the other 49 people will receive no benefit and have to suffer all the adverse effects of the drug because those effects are considered small when compared to the heart attack that the other one person may have.

Such a statistical approach is complete nonsense, and only exists to try to convince doctors that prescribing such drugs to all people is normal and desirable. This is nonsense from a healthcare point of view, because a treatment should always provide a benefit, and it only fails to when the disease mechanism is not understood at all, or the real underlying cause is not understood, so that the intervention then becomes an exercise of taking blind stabs in the dark.

This is like saying that all motor vehicles should be banned because one in every fifty motorists will be involved in an accident at some point in their lives, therefore this ban would theoretically save one in fifty people from having an accident. The problem is that such a

12. Why has an inept, misguided system been adopted by mainstream healthcare?

ban would apply to all people, and the quality of their lives would be diminished because of it (in the same way that the quality of every person's life who takes certain drugs would be diminished, with no positive outcome for them).

The calculation of benefit versus harm

Most common drugs come with long lists of adverse effects; and the role of today's doctors is to manage the damage. Some adverse effects are accepted as a necessary part of the drug-taking process. The patient must just put up with that. It is seen as being in their own best interest. This calculation of "benefit versus harm" is a normal part of a doctor's prescribing process. The drug companies tell them that drugs are "safe and effective." Therefore, the calculation that the patient will be harmed by the drug is a normal train of thought for a doctor, because they have been told the drug is "safe."

For example, with blood-pressure issues, which is one of the commonest prescribing situations, the doctor is simply chasing a number (p.53). The only objective is to get that number to a desired level. In reality, they are unaware of the real underlying issue, so do not address that, leave it in place, and in their goal of "chasing a number", they chemically block the healthy function of a number of aspects of the patient's body, which is then detrimental to all their main organs (p.58). In other words, they have only harmed the patient, and done no good. Yet, due to a doctor's training, and the indoctrination by drug company propaganda, the doctor regards this goal as desirable, and many doctors would be under the delusion that they are doing something to benefit the health of the patient.

Outside of mainstream healthcare, no substance that harms the patient could be considered to be "medicine". By definition, mainstream healthcare does not practice medicine. "Medicine" means a substance used to treat disease. Most drugs are not medicinal because they do not treat a disease. Instead they only chemically block the normal, healthy function of aspects of the body; and do not address the disease (the underlying cause of the symptom) at all. But most doctors would not even be aware of these concepts. From a doctor's point of view, there is no knowledge of how to return organ functions to normal, no knowledge of all the symptoms associated with the subtle organ malfunctions that are produced by simply living in the modern world, and, as far as they know, "medicine" consists of using drugs to chemically block processes in the body. To them, this is normal, and is all there is available. This is the modern, "scientific" approach, and is extensively tested for "safety" and "effectiveness." Or, so a naïve doctor would think (or at least, manage to convince themselves).

The source of information for the media, politicians, and citizens, are doctors, whose source of information is the drug industry (p.91). Hence, this medical religion has spread like no other, and has a deep grasp on the minds of the modern world. But looking at this from outside of the mainstream medical industry, as this book does, mainstream healthcare in its current form is revealed to be probably the biggest and most successful fraud in history. It has a larger following than any religion, and earns billions and billions from the misery it inflicts. I sincerely believe that it is the biggest threat to global healthcare that exists today.

From the people's point of view

If mainstream healthcare is considered a medical religion, what is the extent of that religion's grasp? As an example, during the 2020 respiratory pandemic, which had brought the world to its knees, I never once heard in the media a single commentator pointing out that the whole situation was the result of the ineptitude of mainstream healthcare. The fact is that this is what caused the pandemic. Mainstream healthcare does not have the ability to return an organ to its normal function (in the way that Chinese medicine does routinely). Therefore they could not treat a simple respiratory condition, and everyone became (faithfully, in the nature of religious believers) convinced that it was therefore untreatable, and the only answer was to instead do battle with the pathogen. And in the meantime, they heaped praise on mainstream healthcare (the system that was ruining their lives). Why did people

12. Why has an inept, misguided system been adopted by mainstream healthcare?

have these beliefs, and why did no one notice this great flaw in mainstream healthcare?

This happened because of the belief that if mainstream healthcare could not treat a problem, then it cannot be treated. The faithful all adopted this belief, then dutifully recited the propaganda, that the only answer was to kill the pathogen. Hence, the world became engrossed in the search for a vaccine, reciting another of the main tenets of this medical religion. If we consider the point of view of mainstream healthcare (a relatively new medical religion), this can be compared to the arrogance of youth: if they do not know something, it is considered unknowable. Total faith is ordered, and total faith is given—because the religion is the source of all information, and so, what choice do most people have but to recite the beliefs.

The people are the ultimate victims of all this fraud, but because they trust what they are told by authority figures, the fraud is permitted to flourish. It is true that many people quickly become disillusioned about routine mainstream healthcare—when they have cause to consult it about their routine medical issues. But in general they still turn to a doctor for advice about healthcare matters because that is what the education system has conditioned them to do. And the "science" is easy to understand, and hence can be convincing—to both doctors and patients.

The patient is given a simple equation, which they assume is "scientific". A blood test was performed, and the patient is told that this "shows" a certain thing, and that this proves that they must therefore take a certain drug which will correct the problem. Such an equation is so simple to understand (as simple as "A, B, C"), so it seems convincing—to both patient and doctor. But the patient does not know that the diagnostic test only applies within the limited knowledge of today's physiology. If talking about an organ not functioning correctly, or being "diseased", today's physiology has incomplete knowledge of these matters, which is why it cannot account for how subtle malfunctions in the main organs produce all the common symptoms that people experience due to the normal stresses of living life today (pp.9-13).

Today's physiology's understanding of the organ functions cannot even explain these common mechanisms, so its limited understanding cannot produce a reliable diagnosis. Any diagnosis it makes is based on this incomplete information, but the patient does not know that. They also do not know that mainstream healthcare has no ability to return an organ to its normal function anyway; and that its main tool is to chemically block the normal, healthy function of some other, more superficial aspect of the body, which then also accidentally blocks the function of all the mains organs, preventing them from ever working normally. Most doctors do not appreciate this fact, so it is not surprising that patients do not realize this either.

Instead, the patient's only perception is that they are prescribed some "medication" (and all they understand about "medication" is that it is a "substance" that will make them better—p.31) to tackle a problem that has been identified. They are not in an informed position to make a decision, and so they simply trust what the authority figure tells them.

Another factor in this is human nature. In all areas, people tend to believe what they want to believe, no matter what evidence they are shown. When they have been conditioned their whole life to imagine that doctors are the experts on healthcare, most people would simply believe what a doctor tells them, and ignore all evidence that contradicts this "official" position. Hence, the majority of people tend to blindly follow whatever they are told by mainstream healthcare, and ignore all other information. They are disciples of this medical religion.

The exception usually comes when a person has a health problem that concerns them and they have had a bad experience of mainstream healthcare. Then they have a reason to do all the research necessary to enable them to eventually discover natural healing, in one form or another. From then onwards they tend to be heretics and turn their back on anything offered by mainstream healthcare.

In my experience, there is another class of people. These tend to be genuinely "intelligent" and sensitive people. Often they have already done all the research and thinking necessary to enable them to turn instinctively to natural healing when they have any health problem. In

12. Why has an inept, misguided system been adopted by mainstream healthcare?

my own practice, these patients are always a delight to treat. Because they do not take drug remedies, their bodies respond normally and quickly to treatment, and it is possible to make a big difference to their lives very quickly.

13. What is the value of a diagnosis from mainstream healthcare?

With the knowledge gained from practising and writing about natural healing for over sixteen years, I now tend to automatically mistrust any diagnosis given to a patient by mainstream healthcare. This chapter explains why, gives many examples of such incorrect diagnoses, explains why patients tend to accept such diagnoses, and why the doctor's intervention is usually only damaging to the patient.

In my traditional acupuncture clinic, when I meet a new patient and begin taking their case history, it quickly becomes obvious if the patient is routinely taking pharmaceuticals. With most people, certain of their organs would normally have poor function, and this would produce a range of possible symptoms, with certain symptoms being associated with the poor function of each organ. This could be called the "symptom picture". But when a patient is taking pharmaceuticals, their symptom picture is usually unclear. Many of the expected signs and symptoms that a patient with their conditions would be expected to have, are often not present. The implication is that their organs are being chemically blocked from functioning normally, and hence cannot produce the usual symptoms that are associated with each organ malfunction (pp.9-13).

Hence, when patients are routinely taking drugs, even if they are unaware of the adverse affects, it is clear that their organs are not able to work as they should. Such patients also do not respond well to natural healing. There is an initial response, but then this cannot be maintained. Again, my explanation for this is that because their organs no longer have control over their own chemistry, they are unable to maintain normal function.

It is as though such patients no longer have a human body. And indeed, this is pretty much what is happening. The normal chemistry of their body is suppressed, therefore their body can no longer function in the same way as a "clean" body can. This includes the usual disease mechanisms, as well as the usual state of "normality". I use quotes for "normality" because in today's societies, it is rare for an adult to experience normality for any length of time. Here, I define normality as the state when all their organs are functioning normally, with no symptoms of subtle malfunction being produced, including in their thought patterns and emotions, such as those listed on pages 9-13.

The point here is that most drug interventions do not solve problems; they only prevent a person's organs from ever working normally. Does this mean the diagnoses that led to these interventions were wrong, or were the diagnoses correct, and only the interventions wrong?

Certainly all such drug interventions are wrong, since they do not solve the underlying problem and only cause new problems for the patient in the long run. But in most cases the diagnosis was also wrong, even though superficially it might have made sense and was often even supported by diagnostic tests. I will demonstrate this with some examples.

High blood pressure

Probably the most common reason for drug prescriptions is related to high blood pressure. This was covered in detail in chapters 3 and 4, starting on page 33. Patients have often consulted me with the hope of coming off such drugs. I usually reduce their dose gradually while treating all their organs with acupuncture. In my experience, the more such patients withdraw from such drugs, the more their blood pressure normalises. This suggests that the drugs themselves were also preventing their body from working at a normal blood pressure level (in other words, their organs were prevented from working normally).

It is true that because I treated all their organs with acupuncture, you would expect their blood pressure to become normalized. But the pattern is that the drugs prevent this level being reached, until they are withdrawn completely. That is, even when the person is being treated

13. What is the value of a diagnosis from mainstream healthcare?

with natural healing, the drugs still prevent their organs from returning to normal function for any length of time.

This confirms that the treatment (the drug) was certainly wrong. This is not a big surprise. From the patients I've spoken to, it seems the usual pattern is for their doctor to try them on various different types of drug (Chapter 3), or even combinations of them. Often a drug does not have any effect on their blood pressure (which itself indicates that the theory is incorrect), so a "random" cocktail is tried. And even when the drugs have no real impact on the blood pressure, patients are often left on the drug indefinitely. The mentality of doctors seems to be that "all drugs are safe", so being on such drugs will only, theoretically, be beneficial to the patient, if not now, at some time in the future.

But was the diagnosis wrong? As described in Chapter 3, such a diagnosis is always wrong, because "high blood pressure" is not a disease; it is an indicator that there is a problem somewhere else. But the doctor is not only unaware of the real underlying problem, but most of them (due to their training) have been tricked into thinking that the indicator itself (the high blood pressure) *is* the problem. The response, as described in Chapter 3, is to use a chemical trick to prevent healthy tissue in the body from working normally (either the smooth muscle of blood vessel walls, or even parts of the kidney function), in order to produce a fake impression of lowered blood pressure, and in the process, to accidentally prevent all the main organs from being able to work properly (p.58).

In my experience, when a person is treated with natural healing and all their organs return to normal function, not only do they feel fantastic and enjoy the absence of their previous symptoms, such things as their blood pressure also return to normal. This indicates that the underlying problem was that their organs had previously adopted the habit of working in a constantly stressed state, hence the high blood pressure.

This type of outcome confirms where the true underlying problem lay, and confirms that the number itself (the blood pressure reading) was not the problem. In other words, that it was a wrong approach to chemically block the healthy function of more superficial aspects of

Why Use Natural Healing?

the body in the hope of hiding the problem (or even, that it was wrong to be so medically naive that they thought that that approach *was* tackling the problem).

Asthma, or shortness of breath

In my practice I have encountered many patients who have been prescribed bronchodilator inhalers. This was sometimes for asthma, sometimes for shortness of breath. In all cases, following traditional acupuncture treatment, the patients stopped using the inhalers as they no longer suffered from shortness of breath. In these cases, was the diagnosis wrong, or was the drug wrong?

Asthma is one of the many conditions that mainstream healthcare does not properly understand. Its thinking is that the condition cannot be cured, and that it is caused by swelling of the airways in the lungs.

Both these points are untrue. In cases of asthma where it is hard to breathe in, the underlying cause is poor "kidney" function. This can be easily cured in Chinese medicine by returning the "kidneys" to normal function. When this is done, any asthma (and other conditions related to the "kidneys") will clear immediately, and will remain cured until the poor kidney function returns. In clinic I have often noticed that as soon as I needle a "kidney" acupoint on such a patient, they immediately notice that they can breathe more easily.

Although this association between the "kidneys" and our ability to breathe in has been known for over 2,000 years, mainstream healthcare is unaware of it, which is why they have no idea how to properly treat these conditions.

Note that as mentioned on page 11, when we refer to the "kidneys" in Chinese medicine, this includes three related structures, the kidneys, the adrenal glands and the sex organs. Therefore if mainstream healthcare were to try to investigate the physiology of this relation between the "kidneys" and our ability to breathe in, they would need to look at every aspect of the function of these three structures combined, including the organ communication that is currently unknown to today's physiology (that which takes place in our body via electromagnetic waves).

13. What is the value of a diagnosis from mainstream healthcare?

In asthma patients, mainstream healthcare diagnoses the problem as being a swelling in the smooth muscle of the lung airways. This diagnosis is wrong, since the successful treatment of asthma and many cases of shortness of breath, does not treat those muscles at all, which suggests there is no problem with the lung airways. These are healthy and have normal function. The successful Chinese medicine treatment of asthma suggests that the swelling of the airway muscles is perhaps merely a symptom indicating that the problem is elsewhere (in the patient's "kidney" function). This is confirmed by the fact that when the "kidney" function is treated, the lung airways immediately return to normal function.

Due to this lack of knowledge, the approach of mainstream healthcare is to chemically block the normal function of the smooth muscle that surrounds the lung airways, as described on page 116. This may provide temporary relief, but each time such drugs are used, this weakens the lungs, and always leaves the genuine underlying cause untreated. In some cases, the person's lungs may eventually become so weak that they are unable to function, and the person dies. Page 67 describes the drug industry attempts to cover up the deaths of asthma patients due to inhalers.

In conclusion, the mainstream healthcare diagnosis and treatment are both wrong. And as usual the drug treatment is only damaging in the long term, and does not address the real underlying problem.

All the above also applies to many cases of shortness of breath. But in other cases, the symptom of shortness of breath may be associated with poor heart function. However, in Chinese medicine it has always been known that there is a close functional relationship between the heart and "kidneys". When one of these organs has poor function, the other organ in this pair would usually also be affected, and this may provide an insight into these other cases of shortness of breath.

Depression

I have often successfully treated patients for depression. In Chinese medicine, it is known that the poor function of our main abdominal organs is responsible for directly producing various inappropriate mental and emotional patterns (p.16). With depression, the problem usually lies in the stagnated function of the liver. And once this is corrected with acupuncture treatment, the depression clears, together with any related symptoms, which might include constant anger, irritability, rage, and even violent outbursts.

However, today's healthcare, due to its unawareness of the above mechanisms, assumes that the problem must be in the patient's brain; and they prescribe mind-altering drugs, such as SSRI's. These cause tremendous harm, including agitated states, suicides, and also lethal violence to others, which drug companies have tried to cover up (p.105).

Some of the patients who have consulted me after they were diagnosed as depressed and placed on such anti-depressants, were motivated to seek out natural healing because of the dreadful adverse effects that they experienced.

Of course, the diagnosis of depression is correct if we consider this to be a loose, unspecific description of the patient's condition. But in mainstream healthcare, the diagnosis is that there is something wrong in the person's brain. This is why they attempt to block aspects of the chemistry of the brain. The theory is that SSRI's increase the amount of serotonin in the brain and hence make the person feel better. But this diagnosis is wrong, because the problem does not lie in the brain. Their brain function is normal. The underlying problem lies in the liver function, as demonstrated in Chinese medicine's consistent clinical results. And, as usual, the treatment is also wrong. When drug designers attempt to block normal, healthy functions in the body (in this case, aiming to block it in brain), this only produces many unpredicted adverse effects (due to their knowledge being incomplete); is detrimental to the patient's health; and does not address the real underlying problem.

Anxiety and panic attacks
I have also successfully treated many patients for these conditions. Most of the comments about depression also apply here. But in this case, the underlying cause lies in the heart function. The patient's heart

13. What is the value of a diagnosis from mainstream healthcare?

function will have often been weakened due to events in their personal life. The solution is to return their heart to normal function, which acupuncture achieves immediately; and as long as this normal function is maintained, they no longer experience the anxiety or panic attacks. However, in mainstream healthcare, they do not understand the relationship between our main organs and the whole range of mental and emotional patterns that are produced in us when the associated abdominal organ's function is poor (p.16). This causes them to wrongly imagine that the problem lies in our brain. And since today's biochemistry only has the ability to block normal, healthy function, they attempt to play this trick on the brain's chemistry in order to try to take control of a specific aspect of it (the amount of serotonin, for example), in the hope of correcting what they see as the problem. But this diagnosis and approach to treatment are both wrong and simply cause the patient harm.

Personality disorders

All the above comments also apply in this area. Today's psychiatry has theories about how our mind works, and how common mental and emotional behaviours may be produced in us. But we know this thinking is all misguided, because the actual mechanisms that cause most mental and emotional states were discovered in ancient China (p.16), and this knowledge has produced consistent clinical results ever since.

Due to this misunderstanding, today's psychiatry often invents non-existent conditions (p.101), and prescribes mind-altering drugs to attempt to change the chemistry of a person's brain, when there was nothing wrong with that chemistry in the first place. Needless to say, the patient's health is only impaired by the treatment.

I have even successfully treated such states as extreme agoraphobia by merely returning the key organs to normal function. Due to this Chinese medicine knowledge of how our mental states are produced, and my clinical experiences of how effective acupuncture treatment is in correcting inappropriate mental and emotional states, I now tend to dismiss any notion of "personality disorders" or "chemical imbalances in the brain" that exist in mainstream healthcare. These ideas are misguided, due to their lack of medical knowledge. They are so focused on the microscopic detail that they cannot see basic facts about how the body works.

Hay fever and other allergies

I have successfully treated very many cases of hay fever, often where the patient has had hay fever since childhood and it has had a tremendous negative impact on their life. The treatment has always been to return their "kidney" function to normal, since this is the underlying cause of hay fever, and other allergies. The patients who have experienced this condition since childhood, or for most of their adult lives, find the treatment miraculous, and life transforming.

The "kidneys" in Chinese medicine also includes the adrenal glands, and these organs together are the key organs in providing and maintaining our immunity. This is how the treatment works; it returns the patient's immunity to normal, so that they no longer experience symptoms when exposed to these same pathogens, like pollen, dust, animal fur—just as a person with normal immunity is not affected.

Mainstream healthcare is not aware of this key function of the "kidneys", hence none of their diagnostic tests would be able to detect this particular malfunction in the "kidneys", and they also regard hay fever as having an "unknown" cause.

A normal part of the immune system's response to a pathogen is to produce histamine, which is necessary for a normal immune response. But in the case of a person with hay fever, other elements of their immunity are clearly not working properly. We know this because when the "kidney" function is returned to normal with acupuncture treatment, the person's immunity then works fully and they no longer have hay fever.

However, in mainstream healthcare, most doctors regard hay fever as an allergic reaction. This is a wrong diagnosis. The person is not allergic to pollen; the true problem is that their immune system is not working fully. But as usual, the main option available to drug designers is to chemically block the normal function of some aspect of the body. In this case, they block the production of histamine, with anti-

13. What is the value of a diagnosis from mainstream healthcare?

histamines. Doctors are so used to this way of thinking, that some may even wrongly believe that the production of histamine is the problem.

So, rather than returning the immune system to normal, their approach is to block the aspect of it that was working normally, and leave the real problem unresolved. This does not block the symptoms with all patients, but it can have this effect with some, and, of course, all patients must endure the adverse effects of the drug.

The same is true of other "allergies". These are diagnosed as "allergies", but they are nothing of the sort. The real problem is that the patient's immunity is not working normally. It is true that mainstream healthcare has no idea how to correct the problem, so they do the only thing they know how to, which is to chemically block normal functions in the body, in the hope of concealing the symptoms.

Symptoms related to menstruation

With most women that I have treated, there is a marked improvement in their experience of menstruation. The negative symptoms, such as PMS, period cramps, tender breasts, acne, headaches or migraines, these are all greatly reduced or even cleared completely after a few monthly treatments. The underlying cause in most cases is stagnated liver function. This produces all the symptoms, and also other symptoms, not related to the person's periods, such as general stress and irritability (p.10).

However, mainstream healthcare is unaware of the association of all these symptoms with stagnated liver function; and even if they were aware of the association, they have no ability to return the liver to normal function anyway (since no drug intervention could do this); and they are not even able to detect such a subtle malfunction.

Because of this lack of medical knowledge, when a woman consults a doctor about symptoms related to her period, the usual response is to prescribe hormonal contraceptives with the hope of stopping her periods completely.

This is not so much a wrong diagnosis, as a failure to make a diagnosis at all, due to a lack of medical knowledge. And, as usual, their response chemically blocks a normal, healthy aspect of the body from functioning, in the hope of concealing symptoms, which they have no explanation for. By doing this, they cause all sorts of further complications, some serious. Most hormonal contraceptives weaken the "kidney" function, which can then itself produce a whole range of extra symptoms (p.11), and is certainly seriously detrimental to the person's long-term health.

Muscle and joint pains

In Chinese medicine, there is a detailed knowledge of the "meridians" (p.10). That is, knowledge of which tracts of tissue on the body reflect issues related to a particular organ. When an organ is stressed in any way, this can cause anomalies to appear at certain locations along that organ's related meridian. These anomalies sometimes include stiff or painful joints, or painful muscles. Such joint pains are common at the hips or shoulders. In this case, the underlying cause is in the liver function, and when the liver is returned to normal function with acupuncture treatment, such pains clear immediately. (It is the gallbladder meridian that crosses these locations, but the gallbladder and liver have a close functional relationship, so that problems with the liver function often manifest on the gallbladder meridian.) Similar joint problems can occur at the wrist (related to issues with the lung or heart function) or knees and ankles (usually related to issues with the "kidney" function).

Mainstream healthcare is unaware of these mechanisms, and when joint problems occur, their usual response is to scan the joint, looking for any physical anomalies. If any are found, they assume this is the problem. This is almost always a wrong diagnosis. In my experience, such joint pains can usually be cleared by returning the related organ to normal function. There may well have been a physical anomaly, but this was not the cause of the problem, and any anomaly may also have simply been another reflection of the stress in the related organ. In this case, the anomaly could also gradually clear after the related organ was returned to normal function. In mainstream healthcare, the response is often to resort to surgery, or even to replacing the joint. In comparison to the medical knowledge and sensitivity of Chinese medicine, such an approach is primitive and misguided.

This same situation exists with many types of muscle or tendon pain. This might be diagnosed as RSI or similar. Again, in most instances this is a wrong diagnosis. With the more advanced knowledge of Chinese medicine, it is clear that in many cases, the pain is due to malfunction of the organ associated with the meridian at that location; and the response is to return that organ to normal function, which then clears the pain. In mainstream healthcare, the response may even be to resort to surgery. It is ironical that a medical system from over 2,000 years ago is more sensitive, sophisticated and accurate than today's mainstream healthcare, which, in comparison, may seem like primitive butchery.

Sciatica and neuralgia
I have treated many patients for "sciatica". With these patients they always have stagnated liver function, usually due to stresses in their life. Amongst other symptoms, this also sometimes causes shooting pain down the outside of their upper leg, and sometimes also similar pains elsewhere, centred on the gallbladder and liver meridians. To treat this, I simply return the liver to normal function with acupuncture, which usually happens within the treatment session, clearing the pains, which do not recur until the stress in the person's life has built back up to similar levels, perhaps several months later.

The same mechanism is responsible for producing other pains, such as tingling and deep aching pains at other locations. The explanation for this is that the stressed states in the related organ are being reflected at these bodily locations on the organ's related meridian. And the successful treatment of these pains simply involves returning the organ to normal function with acupuncture. Because the organ is then functioning normally, it is not stressed, so any of the previous pains reflecting that stress, clear.

Mainstream healthcare has no knowledge of this important mechanism, which explains so many of the routine muscular and joint symptoms that people suffer. When a person experiences shooting or tingling pains, the only thing in today's physiology that can possibly account for such pains is improper nerve function, due to damage of some sort. Therefore whenever a doctor considers symptoms such as shooting pains, they always wrongly assume that this must be caused by nerve damage. A common location for this symptom is on the outside of the upper leg, and the nearest nerve to this location is the sciatic nerve. Therefore they assume that the sciatic nerve has a problem, hence their name for this condition is "sciatica."

But this is a wrong diagnosis, arrived at due to a lack of medical knowledge. Part of the gallbladder meridian is situated at this location on the outside of the leg, and this is what is responsible for producing the pain. The tissue along the gallbladder meridian reflects any unusual states in the liver function, so that when the liver is stressed, the tissue at locations along its related meridians also becomes stressed, due to the resonance between the organ and these locations. This mechanism can produce a whole range of symptoms, including shooting pains, tingling, aching, or unusual warmth or redness, or other anomalies. Such anomalies occur in the tissue itself. But the tissue (including the local nerves) is perfectly healthy and there is no local health issue with it.

However, because mainstream healthcare is not aware of these mechanisms, it can only leap to wrong conclusions based on the limit of today's physiology knowledge. Hence it wrongly assumes the cause must be related to nerves, and that a nerve is therefore damaged or "trapped". And, as usual, its intervention can only be damaging to the person's health, since their main tool is to chemically block the normal function of some aspect of the body, which then accidentally impedes the function of the main organs. This does not treat the real underlying condition, in the liver function. The fact is that it would not be able to treat this with drugs anyway, even if it were aware of the real problem, since you cannot return an organ to normal function by chemically blocking the normal, healthy function of any aspect of the body.

The liver and gallbladder meridians exist on many locations on the body, particularly on the head, where many pains are produced by this mechanism. These, of course, are always wrongly diagnosed by mainstream healthcare, due to the above limitations.

13. What is the value of a diagnosis from mainstream healthcare?

Symptoms due to an "infection"

In mainstream healthcare, an "infection" is diagnosed at the drop of a hat, in many different situations. It is almost a kneejerk reaction to any problem, along with their response of prescribing antibiotics. But this is most often a wrong diagnosis.

A common example is the so-called UTI (urinary tract infection). In women, this is usually called thrush. I have treated this condition many times with acupuncture. The cause of the symptoms is an anomaly in the "kidney" and bladder function. When this anomaly is reflected to the meridian locations associated with these organs, it can produce the sensation of burning on urination, itching and soreness. In my experience, such patients always have poor "kidney" function, and when the "kidney" function is returned to normal with acupuncture, the symptoms clear. There are some key acupoints that can clear all these symptoms within seconds; and while the "kidney" function remains at a suitable level, the symptoms do not reappear.

In Chinese medicine, these symptoms are regarded as "heat", which is produced by these organs, and this term is also sometimes used to describe the anomaly in the organs. This "heat", like all organ anomalies, is reflected to the meridian locations associated with these organs, and this is what produces the symptoms at those locations. But this "heat", like much of the ancient Chinese theoretical notions, is a metaphorical description which does not translate to today's terms. And it certainly does not translate to the notion of bacteria. The fact that such symptoms can be cleared within seconds by inserting a needle in the skin at a distance from these symptoms, confirms that the symptoms were not being produced by a bacterial infection.

The same is true of symptoms like ear ache, or a sore throat. These are usually attributed to an "infection". But again, the pain and redness is usually simply reflecting states in the related organ (the "kidneys" and lungs), and when the organ function is returned to normal with acupuncture, these distal symptoms clear, usually within seconds, which itself confirms that there could not have been any "invading bacteria" involved. The symptom of a sore throat being related to a state in the lungs is covered on page 151.

Why Use Natural Healing?

Of course there are bacteria in the throat. These are always present, and are produced within the body as an essential supplement to the immune system activity of clearing dead or foreign cells (p.140). But these bacteria are not "invading" and are not the cause of the sore throat.

There is one slight caveat I would add here. When the distal tissue at any location reflects the stress in the related organ, it is possible that the anomalous state in the distal tissue (which produces the symptoms of redness, pain, itching, etc), may cause our immune system to generate bacteria at that location as a normal part of the immune response. But any such bacteria are not the cause of the anomalous state in the tissue.

This process of an organ's stress being reflected on the skin at key locations on its related meridian, can also commonly produce anomalies in the local tissue and on the skin, such as boils, eruptions, redness, swelling, pain, increased temperate. In mainstream healthcare, these states would normally be diagnosed as an "infection". But this is almost always a wrong diagnosis (see p.150). Today's physiology has no knowledge of the above mechanisms, whereby stress in an organ is reflected to various locations on the body. The only concept in physiology that could be used to explain such symptoms, comes from germ theory, and is the notion that illness in the body is caused by "germs" invading us. This theory has been questioned since it was first suggested (p.140), but it is now used as an explanation for any condition that today's physiology cannot understand.

In this respect, many doctors have adopted the role of ill-informed lay people when it comes to medicine. However, individual doctors are not great thinkers, and they cannot be blamed for acting as they do. They are simply doing what they are told to do (ultimately, by the drug industry, since the whole of mainstream healthcare is led by such commercial concerns). They are priests in a medical religion, and are simply reciting the standard verses.

The verse goes something like this. When there is nothing in today's physiology knowledge that could account for a symptom, the tenets of this religion instruct them to default to this idea that it must be an "infection", and hand out antibiotics. With many such drugs, a doctor's thinking seems to be simply along the lines of "drugs are safe and effective" (because the drug company told us this), so by simply handing out drugs, this will improve a person's health—with no science, logic, or reason at all behind the approach (when analysed by any thinking person). But the reality is that this mainstream medical industry (in its current state) rarely improves the health of the patient (as described throughout this book), and only impedes it in the long run.

Wrongly diagnosed organ "disease"
Today's diagnostic tests are limited by today's physiology knowledge, therefore any conclusion drawn from the tests cannot be taken as reliable.

In general, one of my guiding principles as a healer is that there is nothing inherent in a person's body that dictates they should be diseased. Their physical body is fundamentally normal (in most cases), and any disease present is usually therefore produced by the person's own organs as a response to the routine stresses of life. Therefore any such disease can be cleared by simply clearing their main organs of stress; in other words, returning their organs to normal function.

In many cases, because a physical anomaly is seen in an organ, this does not mean that this cannot be corrected by the organ itself, once it has been returned to normal function with natural healing. The anomaly may be just one more reflection of the stress that the organ is feeling, and like all the anomalies that appear in the tissue at the organ's meridian locations, there is no reason to think that the organ anomalies my not also clear, just as all these distal anomalies do.

But the mainstream healthcare position is to simply imagine the organ is "diseased" and needs to be replaced. I have seen this wrong diagnosis made with the lungs, and a lung transplant became the inevitable outcome of the wrong diagnosis together with the damaging drugs and oxygen given to the patient from that point onwards. But due to my previous examination of the patient, it was clear that the damage to the lungs was due to a bereavement, and I'm certain the condition would have responded to acupuncture treatment, just as I have seen in other patients with similar lung stress. Because the organ stress produces physical anomalies inside the organ, those anomalies are not necessarily the problem. But today's physiology does not understand these common mechanisms; and this limited knowledge compels doctors to leap to wrong conclusions.

Broken bones and wounds

There is one area that mainstream healthcare serves a useful purpose. This is in the common-sense procedures, such as setting a broken bone or stitching up a wound. These areas are common sense because anyone can see what the problem is. It is obvious, therefore the diagnosis is correct. And the intervention does not depend on a knowledge of the microscopic aspects of the body, nor on an attempt to manipulate those. It is a common-sense procedure, so mainstream healthcare is able to adequately perform it.

Conclusion

My experience of natural healing (which was gained from closely studying the ancient classics of Chinese medicine, and practising Chinese acupuncture in clinic for over sixteen years) has provided seemingly profound insights into how our body and mind work and become ill. At least, this knowledge seems profound only when compared to today's physiology, which is unaware of all this knowledge. When considered in its own right, separate from today's mainstream healthcare, the knowledge just seems normal.

The above sections in this chapter describe the common wrong diagnoses that are routinely made by mainstream healthcare, due to the lack of this important medical knowledge. In other words, such diagnoses amount to a self-fulfilling prophecy born from ignorance. Because I am so well versed in natural healing, this brings the inadequate knowledge of mainstream healthcare into sharp focus, and it is this awareness that causes me to tend to dismiss any diagnosis from mainstream healthcare. Add to this the fact that they consider "medicine" to consist of chemically blocking the normal function of aspects of the body, and this destroys any remaining credibility that they might have had as physicians.

References and endnotes

Chapter 3

[1] This includes the communication of organ information on electromagnetic waves, which travel around 670 times faster than nerve impulses, and affect every tissue in our body. This is described in the following paper. Kovich F. What is the Intelligent Tissue Theory and How Does it Relate to Acupuncture? J Acupunct Res 2020;37(4): 241-246. doi: 10.13045/jar.2020.00045.

[2] They used to be called "side effects", but this term was too misleading. It gave the false impression that the drug's design was more informed than it was. In fact, such drugs constitute a more or less random intervention, as evidenced by the vast array of adverse effects which were not predicted and cannot be explained, even by the biochemical engineers who designed the drug.

[3] These adverse effects are taken from the *enalapril* patient information leaflet, and are listed as "common". But the other ACE inhibitors also list similar adverse effects.

[4] Internet source: RxList, 2020. Calcium Channel Blockers (CBCs). A Ogbru, JW Marks. Retrieved from https://www.rxlist.com/calcium_channel_blockers_ccbs/drug-class.htm

[5] Internet source: RxList, 2020. Diuretics. A Ogbru, JW Marks. Retrieved from https://www.rxlist.com/diuretics/drug-class.htm

[6] These known adverse effects were taken from information related to Alfuzosin (Uroxatral). Some other alpha-blockers target different receptors and may include different adverse effects.

Chapter 4

[1] Fletcher Kovich's book, *Acupuncture Today and in Ancient China*, describes this system. And he has also published several papers describing his research into this system. These are summarized at http://www.curiouspages.com/research.

[2] Kovich F. A curious oversight in acupuncture research. J Acupunct Meridian Stud 2017;10(6):411-415. doi: 10.1016/j.jams.2017.10.004.

[3] Internet source: RxList, 2020. High Blood Pressure (Hypertension) Medications. J Morelli, O Ogbru. https://www.rxlist.com/high_blood_pressure_hypertension_medications/drug-class.htm#what_are_the_most_common_blood_pressure_medications

Chapter 5

[1] Weingart SN, Wilson RM, Gibberd RW, et al. Epidemiology of medical error. BMJ. 2000; 320: 774-777.

[2] Starfield B. Is US health really the best in the world? JAMA. 2000; 284: 483-485.

[3] Lazarou J, Pometranz BH, Corey PN. Incidence of adverse drug reactions in hospitalized patients: a meta-analysis of prospective studies. JAMA. 1998; 279: 1200-1205.

[4] Ebbesen J, Buajordet I, Erikssen J, et al. Drug-related deaths in a department of internal medicine. Arch Intern Med. 2001; 161: 2317-2323.

[5] Archibald K, Coleman R, Foster C. Open letter to UK Prime Minister David Cameron and Health Secretary Andrew Lansley on safety of medicines. Lancet. 2011; 377: 1915.

[6] Lenzer J. Anticoagulants cause the most serious adverse events, finds US analysis. BMJ. 2012; 344: e3989.

[7] Brynner R, Stephens T. Dark Remedy: the impact of thalidomide and its revival as a vital medicine. New York: Perseus Publishing; 2001.

[8] Keller MB, Ryan ND, Strober M, et al. Efficacy of paroxetine in the treatment of adolescent major depression: a randomized, controlled trial. J Am Acad Child Adolesc Psychiarty. 2001; 40: 762-72.

[9] Bass A. Side Effects: a prosecutor, a whistleblower, and a bestselling antidepressant on trial. Chapel Hill: Algonquin Books; 2008.

[10] More fraud from drug giant GlaxoSmithKline companies: court documents show. Child Health Safety. 2010 Dec 1.

[11] Moynihan R, Cassels A. Selling Sickness: how the world's biggest pharmaceutical companies are turning us all into patients. New York: Nation Books; 2005.

[12] Peter Gotzsche. Deadly Medicines and Organised Crime: how big pharma has corrupted healthcare. Florida, US: CRC Press, 2017; p.219-222.

[13] Healy G. Let Them eat Prozac. New York University Press; 2004.

[14] Furukawa TA. All clinical trials must be reported in detail and made publically available. Lancet. 2004;329: 626.

[15] Lenzer J. Secret US report surfaces on antidepressants in children. BMJ. 2004; 329: 307.

[16] Lenzer J. Crisis deepens at the US Food and Drug Administration. BMJ. 2004; 329: 1308.

[17] Healy D. SSRI's and deliberate self-harm. Br J Psychiatry. 2002; 180:547.

[18] Khan A, Warner HA, Brown WA. Symptom reduction and suicide risk in patients treated with placebo in antidepressant clinical trials: an analysis of the Food and Drug Administration database. Arch Gen Psychiatry. 2000; 57: 311-17.

[19] Power N, Lloyd K. Response from Pfizer. Br J Psychiatry. 2002; 180: 547-8.

[20] Rockhold F, Mertz A, Traber P. Respone from GlaxoSmithKline. Br J Psychiatry. 2002; 180: 548.

[21] Healy D. Did regulators fail over selective serotonin reuptake inhibitors? BMJ. 2006; 333: 92-5.

[22] Healy D, Cattell D. Interface between authorship, industry and science in the domain of therapeutics. Br j Psychiatry. 2003; 183: 22-7.

[23] Lenzer J. FDA to review 'missing' drug company documents. BMJ. 2005; 330: 7.

[24] Whittington CJ, Kendall T, Fonagy P, et al. Selective serotonin reuptake inhibitors in childhood depression: systematic review of published versus unpublished data. Lancet. 2004; 363: 1341-5.

[25] Seroxat/Paxil Adolescent Depression. Position piece on the phase III clinical studies. GlaxoSmithKline document. 1998 Oct.

[26] Hansson O. Arzneimittel-Multis und der SMON-Skandal. Berlin: Arzneimittel-Informations-Dienst GmbH; 1979.

[27] Knaus H. Corporate profile, Ciba Geigy: pushing pills and pesticides. MultinationalMonitor.org 1993. Internet. https://www.multinationalmonitor.org/hyper/issues/1993/04/mm0493_11.html Accessed 29 Aug 2020.

[28] Dunne M, Flood M, Herxheimer A. Clioquinol: availability and instructions for use. J Antimicrob Chemother. 1976; 2: 21-9.

[29] Pearce N. Adverse Reactions: the fenoterol story. Auckland: Auckland University Press; 2007.

[30] Smith SM, Schroeder K, Fahey T. Over-the-counter (OTC) medications for acute cough in children and adults in ambulatory settings. Cochrane Database Syst Rev. 2008; 1: CD001831.

[31] Gøtzsche Peter. Deadly Medicines and Organised Crime: how big pharma has corrupted healthcare. CRC Press, Florida; 2017: p.14-19.

[32] Gøtzsche PC. Sensitivity of effect variables in rheumatoid arthritis: a meta-analysis of 130 placebo controlled NSAID trials. J Clin Epidemiol. 1990; 43: 1313-18.

[33] Jørgensen FR, Gøtzsche PC, Hein P, et al. [Naproxen (Naprosyn) and mobilization in the treatment of acute ankle sprains]. Ugeskr Læger. 1986; 148: 1266-8.

[34] Rost P. The Whistlebower: confessions of a healthcare hitman. New York: Soft Skull Press; 2006.

[35] Abraham J. Science, Politics and the pharmaceutical industry. London. UCL Press; 1995.

[36] Henry D, Lim LL, Garcia Rodriguez, et al. Variability in risk of gastrointestinal complications with individual non-steroidal anti-inflammatory drugs: results of a collaborative meta-analysis. BMJ. 1996; 312: 1563-6.

[37] Virapen J. Side Effects: death. College Station: Virtualbookworm.com Publishing; 2010.

[38] Joyce C, Lesser F. Opren deaths kept secret, admits Lilly. New Sci. 1985; 107: 15-16.

[39] Cohen D. Complications: tracking down the data on oseltamivir. BMJ. 2009; 339: b5387.

[40] Doshi P. Neuraminidase inhibitors: the story behind the Cochrane review. BMJ. 2009; 339 b5164.

[41] Cohen D. Search for evidence goes on. BMJ. 2012; 344: e458.

[42] Cohen D, Carter P. WHO and the pandemic flu 'conspiracies'. BMJ. 2012; 340: c2912.

[43] Willman D. Relenza: official asks if one day less of flu is worth it. Los Angeles Times. 2000 Dec 20.

[44] Epstein H. Flu warning: beware the drug companies! New York Review of Books. 2001 Apr 11.

[45] Russell J. Johnson & Johnson feels pain of $75m bribery fines. The Telegraph. 2011 Apr 9.

[46] Ark. judge fines Johnson & Johnson more than $1.1B in Risperdal case. CBS/AP. 2012 Apr 11.

[47] Harris G. Research centre tied to drug company. New York Times. 2008 Nov 25.

[48] Kelton E. J&J needs a cure: new CEO allegedly had links to fraud. Forbes. 2012 17 Apr.

[49] Pfizer agrees record fraud fine. BBC News. 2009 Sep 2.

[50] Evans D. Big pharma's crime spree. Bloomberg Markets. 2009 Dec: 72-86.

[51] Rockoff JD, Matthews CM. Pfizer settles federal bribery investigation. Wall Street Journal. 2012 Aug 7.

[52] Barnes K. Sanofi slammed by FDA over failure to act on Ketek fraud. Outsourcing. 2007 Oct 25.

[53] Ross DB. The FDA and the case of Ketek. N Engl J Med. 2007; 356:1601-4.

[54] Soreth J, Cox E, Kweder S et al. Ketek - the FDA perspective. N Eng J Med. 2007; 356: 1675-6.

[55] United States Department of Justice. Novartis Pharmaceuticals Corp. to Pay More than £420 million to Resolve Off-Label Promotion and Kickback Allegations. 2010 Sep 30.

[56] Pringle E. Eli Lilly hides data: Zyprexa, Evista, Prozac risk. ConspiracyPlanet.com

[57] Reuters. The largest pharma fraud whistleblower case in U.S. history totalling $1.4 billion. 2009 Jan 15.

[58] Aventis to pay $95 million to settle fraud charge. AFP. 2009 May 28.

[59] Wikipedia. GlaxoSmithKline. https://en.wikipedia.org/wiki/GlaxoSmithKline.

[60] Carpenter G. Italian doctors face charges over GSK incentive scheme. Over 4000 doctors are alleged to have received cash, gifts, and prizes to encourage them to prescribe GSK products. Lancet. 2004; 363: 1873.

[61] Lane C. Bad medicine: GlaxoSmithKline's fraud and gross negligence. Psychology Today. 2011 Jan 7.

[62] Silverman E. Glaxo to pay $750M for manufacturing fraud. Pharmalot. 2010 Oct 26.

[63] Unite States Department of Justice. GlaxoSmithKline to Plead Guilty and pay $3 billion to resolve Fraud Allegations and Failure to Report Safety Data. 2012 July 2.

[64] Khan H, Thomas P. Drug giant AstraZeneca to pay $520 million to settle fraud case. ABC News. 2010 April 27.

[65] Ibid.

[66] Tanne JH. AstraZeneca pays $520m fine for off-label marketing. BMJ. 2010; 340: c2380.

[67] Silverman E. Merck to pay $670 million over Medicaid fraud. Pharmalot. 2008 Feb 7.

[68] Gansler AG. Abbott Labs to Pay $1.5 Billion More for Medicaid Fraud. Southern Maryland Online. 2012 May 8. http://somd.com/news/headlines/2012/15451.php. Accessed 12 Nov 2020.

[69] Clinard MB, Yeager PC. Corporate Crime. New Brunswick: Transaction Publishers; 2006.

[70] Harris G. As doctor writes prescription, drug company writes a check. New York Times. 2004 Jun 27.

[71] Tanne JH. Bristol-Myers Squibb made to pay $515 m to settle US law suits. BMJ. 2007; 335; 742-3.

[72] Zee A van. The promotion and marketing of OxyContin: commercial triumph, public health tragedy. Am J Publ Health. 2009; 99: 221-7.

[73] Abelson R. Whistle-blower suit says device maker generously rewards doctors. New York Times. 2006 Jan 24.

[74] Poses RM. Medtronic settles, yet again. Health Care Renewal. 2011 Dec 15. https://hcrenewal.blogspot.com/2011/12/medtronic-settles-yet-again.html

[75] Tanne JH. US companies are fined for payments to surgeons. BMJ. 2007; 335: 1065.

[76] Harris G, Pear R. Drug maker's efforts to compete in lucrative insulin market are under scrutiny. New York Times. 2006 Jan 28.

[77] Collier J. Big pharma and the UK government. Lancet. 2006; 367: 97-8.

[78] Ferner RE. The influence of big pharma. BMJ. 2005; 330: 857-8.

[79] Free Online Law Dictionary. Organized crime. https://legal-dictionary.thefreedictionary.com/Organized Crime

[80] Gøtzsche Peter. Deadly Medicines and Organised Crime: how big pharma has corrupted healthcare. CRC Press, Florida; 2017: p.38.

Chapter 6

[1] Marcovitch H. Editors, publishers, impact factors, and reprint income. PLoS Med. 2010; 7: e1000355.

[2] Arroll B, Elley CR, Fishman T, et al. Antidepressants versus placebo for depression in primary care. Cochrane Database Syst Rew. 2009; 3: CD007954.

[3] Hróbjartsson A, Gøtzsche PC. Is the placebo powerless? An analysis of clinical trials comparing placebo with no treatment. N Engl J Med. 2001; 344: 1594-1602.

[4] Hróbjartsson A, Gøtzsche PC. Placebo interventions for all clinical conditions. Cochrane Database Syst Rev. 2010; 1: CD003974.

[5] Gøtzsche Peter. Deadly Medicines and Organised Crime: how big pharma has corrupted healthcare. CRC Press, Florida; 2017: p.44.

[6] Gøtzsche PC. Believability of relative risks and odds ratios in abstracts: cross-sectional study. BMJ. 2006; 333: 231-234.

[7] Hróbjartsson A, Thomsen AS, Emanuelsson F, et al. Observer bias in randomised clinical trials with binary outcomes: systematic review of trials with both blinded and non-blinded outcome assessors. BMJ. 2012; 344: e1119.

[8] Moncrieff J, Wessely S, Hardy R. Active placebos versus antidepressants for depression. Cochrane Database Syst Rev. 2004; 1 : CD003012.

[9] Gøtzsche Peter. Deadly Medicines and Organised Crime: how big pharma has corrupted healthcare. CRC Press, Florida; 2017: p.49.

[10] Gøtzsche PC, Hróbjartsson A, Johansen HK, et al. Constraints on publication rights in industry-initiated clinical trials. JAMA. 2006; 295: 1645-1646.

[11] Speilmans GI, Parry PI. From evidence-based medicine to marketing-based medicine: evidence from internal industry documents. Bioethical Inquiry. 2010. doi:10.1007/s11673-010-9208-8.

[12] Bassler D, Briel M, Montori VM, et al. Stopping randomized trials early for benefit and estimation of treatment effects: systematic review and meta-regression analysis. JAMA. 1020; 303: 1180-1187.

[13] Mello MM, Clarridge BR, Studdert DM. Academic medical centers standards for clinical-trial agreements with industry. N Engl J Med. 2005; 352: 2202-2210.

[14] Steinbrook R. Gag clauses in clinical-trial agreements. N Engl J Med. 2005; 352: 2160-2162.

[15] Chan A-W, Hrøbjartsson A, Haahr MT, et al. Empirical evidence for selective reporting of outcomes in randomized trials: comparison of protocols to published articles. JAMA. 2004; 291: 2457-2465.

[16] Bjelakovic G, Nikolova D, Gluud Li, et al. Antioxidant supplements for prevention of mortality in healthy participants and patients with various diseases. Cochrane Databae Syst Rev. 2008; 2: CD007176.

Chapter 7

[1] Spielmans, G.I., Parry, P.I. From Evidence-based Medicine to Marketing-based Medicine: Evidence from Internal Industry Documents. Bioethical Inquiry 7, 13–29 (2010). doi: https://doi.org/10.1007/s11673-010-9208-8.

[2] Gøtzsche Peter. Deadly Medicines and Organised Crime: how big pharma has corrupted healthcare. CRC Press, Florida; 2017, p74.

[3] Grill M. Kranke Geschäfte: wie die Pharmaindustrie uns manipuliert. Hamburg: Rowohlt Verlag; 2007.

[4] Andersen M, Kragstrup J, Søndergaard J. How conducting a clinical trial affects physicians' guideline adherence and drug preferences. JAMA. 2006; 295: 2759-2764.

[5] Psaty BM, Rennie D. Clinical trial investigators and their prescribing patterns: another dimension to the relationship between physician investigators and the pharmaceutical industry. JAMA. 2006; 295: 2787-2790.

[6] Kassirer JP. On the take: how medicine's complicity with big business can endanger your health. Oxford: Oxford University Press; 2005.

[7] Gøtzsche Peter. Deadly Medicines and Organised Crime: how big pharma has corrupted healthcare. CRC Press, Florida; 2017. Chapter 9, Hard Sell.

[8] Ibid., p.94.

[9] Ibid., pp.87-89.

[10] Moffatt B, Elliott C. Ghost marketing. Perspect Biol Med. 2007; 50:18-31.

[11] Rennie D. When evidence isn't: trials, drug companies and the FDA. J Law Policy. 2007 July: 991-1012.

[12] Gøtzsche Peter. Deadly Medicines and Organised Crime: how big pharma has corrupted healthcare. CRC Press, Florida; 2017, p89-91.

[13] Avorn J, Chen M, Hartley R. Scientific versus commercial sources of influence on the prescribing behaviour of physicians. Am J Med. 1982; 73: 4-8.

[14] Prosser H, Almond S, Walley T. Influences on GPs' decision to prescribe new drugs – the importance of who says what. Fam Pract. 2003; 20: 61-68.

[15] Wazana A. Physicians and the pharmaceutical industry: is a gift ever just a gift? JAMA. 2000; 283: 373-380.

[16] ALLHAT Officers and Coordinators for the ALLHAT Collaborative Research Group. Major outcomes in high-risk hypertensive patients randomized to angiotensin-converting enzyme inhibitor or calcium channel blocker vs diuretic: The antihypertensive and Lipid-Lowering Treatment to Prevent Heart Attack Trial (ALLHAT). JAMA. 2002; 288:2981-2997.

[17] Melander H, Ahlqvist-Rastad J, Meijer G, et al. Evidence b(i)ased medicine – selective reporting from studies sponsored by pharmaceutical industry: review of studies in new drug applications. BMJ. 2003; 326: 1171-1173. doi: 10.1136/bmj.326.7400.1171.

[18] Turner EH, Matthews AM, Linardatos E, et al. Selective publication of antidepressant trials and its influence on apparent efficacy. N Engl J Med. 2008; 358: 252-260.

[19] Rising K, Bacchetti P, Bero L. Reporting bias in drug trials submitted to the Food and Drug Administration: review of publication and presentation PLoS Med. 2008; 5: e217.

[20] Lenzer J. Drug secrets: what the FDA isn't telling. Slate. 2005 Sep 27.

[21] Rennie D. When evidence isn't: trials, drug companies and the FDA. J Law Policy. 2007 July: 991-1012.

[22] Scherer RW, Langenberg P, von Elm E. Full publication of results initially presented in abstracts. Cochrane Database Syst Rev. 2007;2: MR000005.

[23] Gøtzsche PC, Jørgensen AW. Opening up data at the European Medicines Agency. BMJ. 2011; 342: d2686.

[24] Wikipedia. Rimonabant. https://en.wikipedia.org/wiki/Rimonabant#Adverse_effects. Accessed 8 Dec 2020.

[25] Alfter B, Teugels M, Bouma J. Media lift lid on secret reports on drug side-effects. Euobserver. 2008 Oct 22.

[26] Gøtzsche Peter. Deadly Medicines and Organised Crime: how big pharma has corrupted healthcare. CRC Press, Florida; 2017, p.142.

[27] Connolly HM, Crary JL, McGoon MD, et al. Valvular heart disease associated with fenfluramine-phentermine. N Egnl J Med. 1997; 337: 581-588.

[28] Mundy A. Dispensing with the Truth. New York: St. Martin's Press; 2001.

[29] Tansey B. Huge penalty in drug fraud: Pfizer settles felony case in Neurontin off-label promotion. San Francisco Chronicle. 2004 May 14.

[30] Lenzer J. Pfizer pleads guilty, but drug sales continue to soar. BMJ. 2004; 328: 1217.

[31] Angell M. The Truth about the Drug Companies: how they deceive us and what to do about it. New York: Random House; 2004.

[32] Petersen M. Suit says company promoted drug in exam rooms. New York Times. 2002 May 15.

[33] Gøtzsche Peter. Deadly Medicines and Organised Crime: how big pharma has corrupted healthcare. CRC Press, Florida; 2017. p.152.

[34] Voris B, Lawrence J. Pfizer Told to Pay $142.1 million for Neurontin Fraud. Bloomberg. 2010 Mar 25.

[35] Adams C, Young A. Off-label prescriptions case reflects federal concern over unsafe uses. Knight Ridder Newspapers. 2004 May 14.

[36] Krumholz HM, Ross JS, Presler AH, et al. What have we learned from Vioxx? BMJ. 2007; 334:120-123.

[37] Topol EJ. Failing the public health – rofecoxib, Merck, and the FDA. N Engl J Med. 2004; 351: 1707-1709.

[38] Weaver AL, Messner RP, Storms WW, et al. Treatment of patients with osteoarthritis with rofecoxib compared with nabumetone. J Clin Rheumatol. 2006; 12: 17-25.

[39] Bombardier C, Laine L, Reicin A, et al. Comparison of upper gastrointestinal toxicity of rofecoxib and naproxen in patients with rheumatoid arthritis. N Engl J Med. 2000; 343: 1520-1528.

[40] Gøtzsche Peter. Deadly Medicines and Organised Crime: how big pharma has corrupted healthcare. CRC Press, Florida; 2017, p.156.

[41] Charatan F. 94% of patients suing Merck over rofecoxib agree to terms. BMJ. 2008; 336: 580-581.

[42] Berenson A. Merck agrees to settle Vioxx suits for $4.85 billion. New York Times. 2007 Nov 9.

[43] Department of Justice. U.S. pharmaceutical company Merck Sharp & Dohme sentenced in connection with unlawful promotion of Vioxx. 2012 April 19.

[44] Jørgensen AW, Jørgensen KJ, Gøtzsche PC. Unbalanced reporting of benefits and harms in abstracts on rofecoxib. Eur J Clin Pharmacol. 2010; 66: 341-347.

[45] Gøtzsche Peter. Deadly Medicines and Organised Crime: how big pharma has corrupted healthcare. CRC Press, Florida; 2017, p.160-162.

[46] Thomas K. In documents on pain drug Celebrex, signs of doubt and deception. New York Times. 2012 Jun 24.

[47] Gøtzsche Peter. Deadly Medicines and Organised Crime: how big pharma has corrupted healthcare. CRC Press, Florida; 2017. p164.

[48] Silverstein FE, Faich G, Goldstein JL, et al. Gastrointestinal toxicity with celecoxib vs nonsteroidal anti-inflammatory drugs for osteoarthritis and rheumatoid arthritis: the CLASS study: A randomized controlled trial. Celecoxib Long-term Arthritis Safety Study. JAMA. 2000; 284: 1247-1255.

[49] Jüni P, Rutjes AW, Dieppe PA. Are selective COX 2 inhibitors superior to traditional non steroidal anti-inflammatory drugs? BMJ. 2002; 324: 1287-1288.

[50] Lu HL. Statistical Reviewer Briefing Document for the Advisory Committee. FDA. 2000; NDA20-998.

[51] Abramson J. Overdo$ed America. New York: HarperCollins; 2004.

[52] Solomon SD, McMurry JJ, Pfeffer MA, et al. Cardiovascular risk associated with celecoxib in a clinical trial for colorectal adenoma prevention. N Engl J Med. 2005; 352: 1071-1080.

[53] Caldwell B, Aldington S, Weatherall M, et al. Risk of cardiovascular events and celecoxib: a systematic review and meta-analysis. J R Soc Med. 2006; 99: 132-140.

[54] Gøtzsche Peter. Deadly Medicines and Organised Crime: how big pharma has corrupted healthcare. CRC Press, Florida; 2017. p.167.

[55] Mamdani M, Juurlink DN, Kopp A, et al. Gastrointestinal bleeding after the introduction of COX 2 inhibitors: ecological study. BMJ. 2004; 328: 1415-1416.

[56] Blower AL, Brooks A, Fenn GC, et al. Emergency admissions for upper gastrointestinal disease and their relation to NSAID use. Aliment Pharmacol Ther. 1997; 11: 283-291.

[57] Cohen D. Rosiglitazone: what went wrong? BMJ. 2010; 341: 530-534.

[58] Harris G. Diabetes drug maker hid test data. New York Times. 2010 Jul 13.

[59] Bass A. Side effects – a prosecutor, a whistleblower, and a bestselling antidepressant on trial. Chapel Hill: Algonquin Books; 2008.

[60] Nissen SE, Wolski K. Effect of rosiglitazone on the risk of myocardial infarction and death from cardiovascular causes. N Engl J Med. 2007; 356: 2457-2471.

[61] Nissen SE. Setting the RECORD straight. JAMA. 2010; 303: 1194-1195.

[62] Moynihan R. Rosiglitazone, marketing, and medical science. BMJ. 2010; 340: c1884.

Chapter 8

[1] Moynihan R, Cassels A. Selling Sickness: how the world's biggest pharmaceutical companies are turning us all into patients. New York: Nation Books; 2005.

[2] IMS Health. IMS Health Reports US prescription Sales Grew 5.1 percent in 2009, to $300.3 billion. Press release. 2010 Apr 1.

[3] Spence D. The psychiatric oligarchs who medicalise normality. BMJ. 2012; 344: e3135.

[4] Gross J. Checklist for camp: bug spray, sunscreen, pills. New York Times. 2006 Jul 16.

[5] Whitaker R. Anatomy of an Epidemic. New York: Broadway Paperbacks; 2010.

[6] Morbidity and Mortality Weekly Report. Current depression among adults – United States, 2006 and 2008. JAMA. 2010; 304: 2233-2235.

[7] Gøtzsche Peter. Deadly Medicines and Organised Crime: how big pharma has corrupted healthcare. CRC Press, Florida; 2017, page 194.

[8] Healy D. Let Them Eat Prozac. New York: New York University Press; 2004.

[9] Friedman RA. Grief, depression, and the DSM-5. N Engl J Med. 2012; 366: 1855-1857.

[10] Nielsen M, Gøtzsche P. An analysis of psychotropic drug sales. Increasing sales of selective serotonin reuptake inhibitors are closely related to number of products. Int J Risk Saf Med. 2011; 23: 125-132.

[11] Larson JC, Ensrud KE, Reed SD, et al. Efficacy of escitalopram for hot flashes in healthy menopausal women: a randomised controlled trial. JAMA. 2011; 305: 267-274.

[12] Coupland C, Dhiman P Morriss R, et al. Antidepressant use and risk of adverse outcomes in older people: population based cohort study. BMJ. 2011; 343: d4551.

[13] Whitaker R. Anatomy of an Epidemic. New York: Broadway Paperbacks; 2010.

[14] Gøtzsche Peter. Deadly Medicines and Organised Crime: how big pharma has corrupted healthcare. CRC Press, Florida; 2017, p.191.

[15] Moore TJ, Glenmullen J, Furberg CD. Prescription drugs associated with reports of violence towards others. PLoS One. 2010; 5: e15337.

[16] Gøtzsche Peter. Deadly Medicines and Organised Crime: how big pharma has corrupted healthcare. CRC Press, Florida; 2017, p.202

[17] Jakobsen, J.C., Katakam, K.K., Schou, A. et al. Selective serotonin reuptake inhibitors versus placebo in patients with major depressive disorder. A systematic review with meta-analysis and Trial Sequential Analysis. BMC Psychiatry 17, 58 (2017). https://doi.org/10.1186/s12888-016-1173-2

[18] Montejo A, Llorca G, Izquierdo J, et al. Incidence of sexual dysfunction associated with antidepressant agents: a prospective multicentre study of 1022 outpatients. Spanish Working Group for the study of psychotropic-related sexual dysfunction. J Clin Psychiatry. 2001: 62 (Suppl.3):10-21

[19] Healy D. Let Them Eat Prozac. New York: New York University Press; 2004

[20] Gøtzsche Peter. Deadly Medicines and Organised Crime: how big pharma has corrupted healthcare. CRC Press, Florida; 2017, p.203

[21] Virapen J. Side Effects: death. College Station: Virtualbookworm.com Publishing; 2010.

[22] Teicher MH, Gold C, Cole JO. Emergence of intense suicidal preoccupation during fluoxetine treatment. Am J Psychiatry. 1990; 147: 207-210

[23] Healy D. Pharmageddon. Berkeley: University of California Press; 2012.

[24] Lenzer J. FDA to review 'missing' drug company documents. BMJ. 2005; 330:7.

[25] Gøtzsche Peter. Deadly Medicines and Organised Crime: how big pharma has corrupted healthcare. CRC Press, Florida; 2017, p.205.

[26] Lenzer J. Drug secrets: what the FDA isn't telling. Slate. 2005 Sep 27.

[27] Lenzer J. Secret US report surfaces on antidepressants in children. BMJ. 2004; 329: 307.

[28] Whitaker R. Anotomy of an Epidemic. New York: Broadway Paperbacks; 2010.

[29] Boseley S. They said it was safe. The Guardian. 1999 Oct 30.

[30] Jurand SH. Lawsuits over antidepressants claim the drug is worse than the disease. American Association for Justice. 2003 Mar 1.

[31] Babyak M, Blumenthal JA, Herman S, et al. Exercise treatment for major depression: maintenance of therapeutic benefit at 10 months. Psychosom Med. 2000 Sep-Oct; 62: 633-638.

[32] Haug TT, Blomhoff S, Hellstrøm K, et al. Exposure therapy and sertraline in social phobia: 1-year follow-up of a randomised controlled trial. Br J Psychiatry. 2003; 182: 312-318.

[33] Herxheimer A. Turbulence in UK medicines regulation: A stink about SSRI antidepressants that isn't going away. Galvanis K, O'Donovan O, editors. Power, Politics and Pharmaceuticals: drug regulation in Ireland in the global context. Cork: Cork university Press; 2008.

[34] Medawar C, Hardon A. Medicines out of Control? Antidepressants and the conspiracy of goodwill. Netherlands: Aksant Academic Publishers; 2004.

[35] Gøtzsche Peter. Deadly Medicines and Organised Crime: how big pharma has corrupted healthcare. CRC Press, Florida; 2017, p 210-211.

Chapter 9

[1] Gilbert, N. Regulations: Herbal medicine rule book. Nature 480, S98–S99 (2011). https://doi.org/10.1038/480S98a.

[2] World Health Organization. Editor Dr Xiaorui ZHANG, Traditional Medicine Programme. Regulatory Situation of Herbal Medicines A worldwide Review. WHO/TRM/98.1. 1998.

[3] Miller LH, Su X. Artemisinin: discovery from the Chinese herbal garden. Cell. 2011;146(6):855-858. doi:10.1016/j.cell.2011.08.024

[4] Gøtzsche Peter. Deadly Medicines and Organised Crime: how big pharma has corrupted healthcare. CRC Press, Florida; 2017, p.202.

[5] Zadronzy B. Amazon removes books promoting autism cures and vaccine misinformation. NBC News. Mar 13 2019. https://www.nbcnews.com/tech/internet/amazon-removes-books-promoting-autism-cures-vaccine-misinformation-n982576

[6] SS An, TR Bai, JHT Bates, et al. Airway smooth muscle dynamics: a common pathway of airway obstruction in asthma. European Respiratory Journal 2007 29: 834-860; doi: 10.1183/09031936.00112606

[7] Kovich F. Acupuncture Today and in Ancient China. Bristol, United Kingdom: CuriousPages Publishing, 2019, Chapters 2-3.

Chapter 10

[1] Mortimer, E. Pertussis Immunization. Hospital Practice, 1980; October: 103.

[2] Dubos R. Mirage of Health. Harper, 1959, p.73.

[3] Bernard Harris & Jonas Helgertz (2019) Urban sanitation and the decline of mortality, The History of the Family, 24:2, 207-226, doi: 10.1080/1081602X.2019.1605923.

[4] Gallardo - Albarrán, D. (2020), Sanitary infrastructures and the decline of mortality in Germany, 1877 – 1913†. The Economic History Review, 73: 730-757, doi: 10.1111/ehr.12942.

[5] Ivan I. Medical Nemesis: The expropriation of health. Pantheon Books, New York; 1976.

[6] Dubos, R., Mirage of Health, Harper, 1959, p.74-75.

[7] Stewart GT. Vaccination Against Whooping Cough: Efficacy versus Risks. The Lancet, 1977;309(8005):234-237. doi: 10.1016/S0140-6736(77)91028-5.

[8] Mendelsohn R. The Truth About Immunizations. The People's Doctor, 1978; April:1.

[9] Cherry J. The New Epidemiology of Measles and Rubella. Hospital Practice; July 1980, p.52-54.

[10] HR 10541. cited by Trebing WP. Good-bye Germ Theory: ending a century of medical fraud and how to protect your family. Xlibris Corporation; 2006.

[11] Trebing WP. Good-bye Germ Theory: ending a century of medical fraud and how to protect your family, 6th edition. Xlibris, 2006, p.124.

[12] Ibid., p.121.

[13] Dang-Tan T, M Mahmud S, Puntoni R. et al. Polio vaccines, Simian Virus 40, and human cancer: the epidemiologic evidence for a causal association. Oncogene 23, 6535–6540 (2004). doi: 10.1038/sj.onc.1207877.

[14] Trebing WP. Good-bye Germ Theory: ending a century of medical fraud and how to protect your family, 6th edition. Xlibris, 2006, p.126.

[15] Ibid., p.120.

[16] Ibid., p.118.

[17] Stewart G. Vaccination Against Whooping Cough: Efficiency vs. Risks. Lancet, 1977; p.234.

[18] Family Practice News; 1980; July 15, p.1.

[19] Ferrante J. Atypical Symptoms? It Could Still Be Measles. Modern Medicine; 1980; Sep 30: 76.

[20] Cherry J. The New Epidemiology of Measles and Rubella. Hospital Practice; 1980; July: 53.

[21] Davis B, et al. Microbiology, 2nd Ed. Harper, 1973; p.1418.

[22] Hayflick L. Slow Viruses. Executive Health Report, 1981; Feb: 1-4.

[23] Davis B, et al. Microbiology, 2nd Ed. Harper, 1973: 1418-1449.

[24] Mendelsohn R. The Truth About Immunizations. The People's Doctor, April 1978, p.1.

[25] Trebing WP. Good-bye Germ Theory: ending a century of medical fraud and how to protect your family, 6th edition. Xlibris, 2006, p.134.

[26] Ibid., p.135.

[27] Ibid., pp.136-141.

[28] Ibid., p.140.

[29] Information taken from the Prescribing Information leaflet for Sanofi Pasteur Full 253 – DAPTACEL.

[30] Trebing WP. Good-bye Germ Theory: ending a century of medical fraud and how to protect your family, 6th edition. Xlibris, 2006, p.67.

[31] Wikipedia. Robert S Mendelsohn. https://en.wikipedia.org/wiki/Robert_S._Mendelsohn.

[32] Trebing WP. Good-bye Germ Theory: ending a century of medical fraud and how to protect your family, 6th edition. Xlibris, 2006, p.73.

[33] Ibid., p.76.

[34] Ibid., p.120.

[35] Ibid., p.193.

[36] Brown P. Illegal vaccine link to Gulf war syndrome. The Gaurdian, 2001; 30 Jul. https://www.theguardian.com/environment/2001/jul/30/internationalnews.

[37] Trebing WP. Good-bye Germ Theory: ending a century of medical fraud and how to protect your family, 6th edition. Xlibris, 2006, p.169.

[38] Ibid., p.151.

[39] Ibid., p.154.

[40] Verner JR, Weiant CW, Watkins RJ. Rational Baceriology. Self published, 1953. To obtain a copy, see https://soilandhealth.org/copyrighted-book/rational-bacteriology.

References and endnotes

Chapter 11

[1] Kovich F. How Our Body's Evolution was guided by Our Abdominal Organs (The Intelligence behind Evolution). Insights Anthropol 2020; 4(2):290-293. doi:10.36959/763/513.

[2] Kovich F. Acupuncture Today and in Ancient China. Bristol, United Kingdom: CuriousPages Publishing, 2019, p.308.

[3] Kovich F. How Our Body's Evolution was guided by Our Abdominal Organs (The Intelligence behind Evolution). Insights Anthropol 2020; 4(2):290-293. doi: https://doi.org/10.36959/763/513.

[4] Kovich F. What is the Intelligent Tissue Theory and How Does it Relate to Acupuncture? J Acupunct Res 2020;37(4): 241-246. doi: 10.13045/jar.2020.00045.

[5] Kovich F. Hernia treated with acupuncture, case history. CuriousPages.com, 21 July 2016. http://www.curiouspages.com/sketchbook/TCMherniaTreatedWithAcupuncture.php.

Index

Abbott, 76
abdominal bloating, 9
ACE inhibitor, 37, 53
acne, 183
ADHD, 102
adrenal glands, 21
Advair, 74
agammaglobulinemia, 132
AIDS, 133
allergic reaction, 182
allergies, 11, 183
ALLHAT, 91
Alpha-beta blockers, 48
Alpha-blockers, 45
alzheimer's, 75
Alzheimer's, 73
Angell, Marcia, 79
anger, 180
angiotensin converting enzyme, 37
angiotensin II, 37
Angiotensin II receptor blockers, 40
antioxidants, 88
anxiety, 13, 75, 180
apathy, 12
aphasia, 13
appetite, 9, 39
ARB's, 40
Artemisia annua, 112
artemisinin, 112

asthma, 12, 116, 178
Astra-Syntex, 68
AstraZeneca, 75, 85, 90
atypical diseases, 131
atypical measles, 131
Avandia, 74, 98
AZT, 133
Bechamp, Pierre, 140
benazepril, 38
benoxaprofen, 69
Beta-blocker, 41
Bextra, 71
Biomet, 77
blood pressure, 33, 176
BMJ, 69
Boehringer Ingelheim, 68
Bristol-Myers Squibb, 76, 85
bruise easily, 9
bubonic plague, 141
Calcium channel blockers, 42
Capoten, 38
captopril, 38
CCBs, 42
Celebrex, 97
Chinese herbal medicine, 111
Chinese medicine, 9, 49, 145
cholera, 123
Ciba, 67
Cipralex, 103
Clenner, Dr Fred, 124
clioquinol, 67

constipation, 11
controlling, 11, 17
cough, 12, 39
cramps, 10
Craten, Dr Charles, 126
Creutzfeldt-Jakob disease, 131
Cymbalta, 107
deafness, 11
Defeating Personality Disorder, 101
dementia, 12, 73, 75
Depakote, 76
depression, 11, 13, 73, 75, 179
DePuy Orhopaedics, 77
Diagnostic and Statistical Manual of Mental Disorders, 101
Dickersin, Kay, 95
diphtheria, 123, 124, 128
Diuretics, 44
dizziness, 11
double blind, 82
DPT, 137, 138
DSM, 101, 102
Dubos, René, 123
Duesberg, Dr Peter, 133
duloxetine, 107
dyslexia, 13
easily startled, 13
Eli Lilly, 69, 73, 101, 105
EMA, 93
emotional fluctuations, 11
enalapril, 38
encephalopathy, 128
escitalopram, 103

European Medicines Agency, 93
Evista, 73
excess gas, 9
FDA, 65, 70, 71, 72, 74, 92, 94, 96, 97, 137, 139
fearful, 11
Feldene, 69
fenoterol, 68
Fen-Phen, 93
Flonase, 74
fluoxetine, 63, 105
food intolerance, 9
frequent urination, 11
Geodon, 71
Glaxo, 64, 98
GlaxoSmithKline, 63, 70, 74, 108
Gøtzsche, Peter, 65, 81, 93
Greenburg, Dr Bernard, 124
grief, 23
Grünenthal, 62
Guillain-Barré syndrome, 131
haemorrhages, 9
hay fever, 11, 182
headache, 39, 114, 183
Healy, David, 65
herbal remedies, 32
herpes simplex, 131
hiccup, 10
HIV, 133
hot flushes, 12, 103
hysteria, 13
IBS, 18, 114, 156
impotence, 12

incontinence, 11
infection, wrong diagnosis, 187
infertility, 12
inhaler deaths, 67
insomnia, 11, 12, 13
intelligent tissue theory, **153**, 165
introverted, 13
Irbesartan, 40
irritability, 10, 11, 180
isoprenaline, 68
Janssen, 71, 85
Johnson & Johnson, 71
joint pain, 184
Keller, Martin, 64
Ketex, 72
kuru, 131
Lamictal, 74
lethargy, 13
leukocytopenia, 133
Lexapro, 103
Liam Grant, 93
libido, 21
lightheaded feeling, 11
Lilly, 66, 85
lisinopril, 38, 53
loose stools, 9, 11
Lundbeck, 103
Lyrica, 71
malaria, 112
Masochistic Personality Disorder, 101
Massachusetts Department of Mental Health, 64
measles, 124, 127, 128, 129
Medtronic, 77
melancholy, 11
Mendelsohn, Dr Robert S, 137
menstruation, 9, 114, 183
Merck, 75, 96
meridian, 10, 15
Microzyma, 140
migraines, 11, 114, 183
mumps, 131
muttering, 13
Naprosyn, 68
naproxen, 68
neuralgia, 185
Neurontin, 94, 95
New England Journal of Medicine, 79
night sweating, 12
NNT, 168
North Carolina Health Dept, 124
Novartis, 67, 72
NSAID, 68, 97
number needed to treat, 168
oedema, 11
Oppositional Defiant Disorder, 101
Opren, 69
Oraflex, 69
ovarian cancer, 73
Oxactin, 63
OxyContin, 76
P value, 80, 161
palpitations, 13
pancreas, 9
pandemic, 114, 149, 170

panic attacks, 13, 180
paracetamol, 64
paranoia, 11, 13
paroxetine, 63, 98
Pasteur, Louis, 129, 140
Paxil, 63, 74, 108
Pearce, Neil, 68
perfectionist, 23
period cramps, 183
personality disorder, 181
pertussis, 123, 128
Pfizer, 65, 66, 69, 71, 72, 89, 94, 95, 97
Pharmacia, 97
phentermine, 93
Philippines, 127
piroxicam, 69
placebo effect, 79, 162
PMS, 11, 183
polio, 124
poliomyelitis, 123, 125
Pondimin, 93
premature ejaculation, 11
Premenstrual Dysphoric Disorder, 101
Prinivil, 53
protocol, drug trial, 86
Prozac, 63, 101, 104, 105
pulses, 15
Purdur Pharma, 76
rabies, 129
Racketeer Influenced and Corrupt Organizations Act, 77
rage, 180

ramipril, 38
RICO, 77, 95
Riker, 68
Risperdal, 71
Roaccutane, 93
Roche, 70, 93
rosiglitazone, 98
RSI, 185
Salk, Jonas, 126
Sanofi-Aventis, 72, 73, 93
saprophytes, 141
scarlet fever, 128
sciatica, 185
seeding trials, 105
selective serotonin reuptake inhibiter, 63
self-preservation, 21
senility, 12
Sereoxat, 108
Serono Laboratories, 77
Seroquel, 75
Serostim, 77
serotonin, 104
Seroxat, 63
sertraline, 108
sex organs, 21
Shaw, George Bernard, 127
shingles, 131
short term memory, 12
shortness of breath, 12, 13, 39, 178
SIDS, 137
sighing, 10
Simian Virus 40, 126
sinuses, 12

Index

small pox, 126
smell, sense of, 12
Smith & Nephew, 77
SmithKline Beecham, 98, 108
social phobia, 108
speech defects, 13, 20
SSPE, 132
SSRI, 63, 92, 103, 108, 180
stammering, 13, 20
statistically significant, 81
stress, 15
Stryker Orthopaedics, 77
stuttering, 13, 20
subacute sclerosing panencephalitis, 132
Sudden Infant Death Syndrome, 137
suicides concealed, 66
SV40, 126
sweating, spontaneous, 13
Takeda, 76
Tamiflu, 70
TAP Pharmaceuticals, 76, 90
taste, 39
taste, sense of, 9
TB, 123, 128
Teicher, Martin, 106
tender breasts, 11, 183
tetanus, 123
thalidomide, 62
thought patterns produced by organs, 16
tinnitus, 11
tongue examination, 14
Toshi Furukawa, 66

Trileptal, 72
tumors, 132
typhoid, 123
typhus, 123
UK, 63, 98, 104, 128
US Centres for Disease Control, 101
US Food and Drug Administration. *See FDA*
vaccination, 123
vaccination theory, 129
VAERS, 139
vancomycin, 72
vasodilator, 37
Vasotec, 38
vertigo, 11
Vilchez, RA, 126
Vioxx, 96
visual disturbances, 11
Warner-Lambert, 94
warts, 131
weakness, 9
Wellbutrin, 74
whooping cough, 123, 124, 128
worrying, 19
Wyeth, 93, 138
zanamivir, 70
Zestril, 53
Zimmer, 77
Zoladex, 75
Zoloft, 108
Zyprexa, 73
Zyvox, 71

Further reading

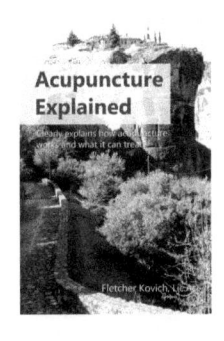

Acupuncture Explained
Fletcher Kovich
This inexpensive book enables the general reader to fully understand what acupuncture is, how it works and what it can treat. It enables you to understand every aspect of the treatment and your condition, including any mental or emotional cause.

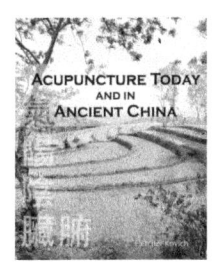

Acupuncture Today and in Ancient China
Fletcher Kovich
This book is a substantial textbook. It provides all the content of the above book, but with much greater detail on the history and the progression of Chinese medicine acupuncture from its earliest roots. Also included are references to all the ancient source material, and details of the latest research on how acupuncture works.

The following papers may also be downloaded free of charge:

Kovich F. How Our Body's Evolution was guided by Our Abdominal Organs (The Intelligence behind Evolution). Insights Anthropol 2020; 4(2):290-293. doi: 10.36959/763/513

Kovich F. What is the Intelligent Tissue Theory and How Does it Relate to Acupuncture? J Acupunct Res 2020;37(4): 241-246. doi: 10.13045/jar.2020.00045

Please visit **www.curiouspages.com/books** for details of free sample downloads, full details of the above books, and a complete list of books available.